IMMUNOMODULATION BY INTRAVENOUS IMMUNOGLOBULIN

Organizing Committee

R. Dierdorf
A. Morell
E. A. Oswald
E. Rewald
H. Sinclair
P. Wormser

IMMUNOMODULATION
BY INTRAVENOUS
IMMUNOGLOBULIN

The Proceedings of a Symposium held at the
24th Congress of the International Society of Haematology,
London, UK, August 1992, combined with the Proceedings of an
International Symposium held in Mar del Plata, Argentina,
October 1992

EDITED BY
E. REWALD AND A. MORELL

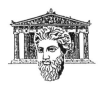

The Parthenon Publishing Group
International Publishers in Medicine, Science & Technology

Casterton Hall, Carnforth,
Lancs LA6 2LA, UK

One Blue Hill Plaza, PO Box 1564
Pearl River, New York 10965, USA

Published in the UK and Europe by
The Parthenon Publishing Group Limited
Casterton Hall, Carnforth,
Lancs. LA6 2LA, England

Published in the USA by
The Parthenon Publishing Group Inc.
One Blue Hill Plaza,
Pearl River,
New York 10965, USA

ISBN: 1-85070-510-0

British Library Cataloguing in Publication Data
Immunomodulation by Intravenous
Immunoglobulin: Proceedings of a Symposium
Held at the 24th Congress of the
International Society of Haematology,
London, UK, August 1992, Combined with
the Proceedings of an International Symposium
Held in Mar del Plata, Argentina, October, 1992
  I. Rewald, E. II. Morell, A.
  616.079
    ISBN 1-85070-510-0

Library of Congress Cataloging-in-Publication Data
International Society of Hematology. Congress, 24th (1992: London,
  England)
    Immunomodulation of intravenous immunoglobulin: the proceedings
  of a symposium held at the 24th Congress of the International
  Society of Haematology, London, UK, August 1992, combined with the
  proceedings of an international symposium held in Mar del Plata,
  Argentina, October 1990 / edited by E. Rewald and A. Morell.
      p. cm.
    Includes bibliographical references and index.
    ISBN 1-85070-510-0
    1. Immunoglobulins—Therapeutic use—Congresses. I. Rewald, E.
  II. Morell, A. (Andreas) III. Title.
    [DNLM: 1. Immunoglobulins, Intravenous—therapeutic use-
  -congresses. QW 601 I6127i 1992]
  RM282.I44I58 1992
  615'.37—dc20
  DNLM/DLC   93-19427
  for Library of Congress   CIP

Typeset by Blackpool Typesetting Services Ltd., Blackpool
Printed and bound in Great Britain by
Butler & Tanner Ltd., Frome and London

Contents

Contents

List of principal contributors

M. Basta
National Institutes of Health
Laboratory of Clinical Investigation
Building 10, Room 11 N 228
9000 Rockville Pike
Bethesda, Maryland 20892
USA

F. Benaim
School of Burns and Repair Surgery
  of Burn Sequels
Universidad del Salvador
Buenos Aires
Argentina

M. A. Boogaerts
University Hospital
3000 Leuven
Belgium

H. Borberg
Haemapheresis
Department of Medicine
University of Köln
Joseph-Stelzmann-Strasse 9
D-5000 Köln-Lindenthal 41
Germany

E. Bullorsky
Hospital Britanico (Hematologia)
Pedriel 74(1280)
Buenos Aires
Argentina

M. M. S. Carneiro-Sampaio
Department of Immunology
Universidade de São Paulo
05508-900 São Paulo
Brazil

H. Cottier
Institute of Pathology
University of Berne
Murtenstrasse 31
CH 3010 Berne
Switzerland

C. B. Coulam
Genetics and IVF Institute
3020 Javier Road
Fairfax
Virginia 22031
USA

L. Dominioni
Department of Surgery
University of Pavia
Ospedale Multizonale
21100 Varese
Italy

J. M. Dwyer
Department of Clinical Immunology
Prince Henry/Prince of Wales
  Hospitals of the University of
  New South Wales School of
  Medicine
Sydney
Australia

E. W. Gelfand
National Jewish Center for
  Immunology and Respiratory
  Medicine
1400 Jackson Street
Denver
Colorado 80206
USA

B. González Martín
Division of Clinical Immunology
Hospital Luis Calvo Mackenna
Santiago
Chile

A. Hässig
Sonneggweg 4
CH-3066 Stettlen
Switzerland

P. A. Imbach
Children's Hospital Aarau and Basle
University of Basle
4005 Basle
Switzerland

S. V. Kaveri
Hôpital Broussais
96 Rue Didot
75014 Paris
France

M. D. Kazatchkine
Hôpital Broussais
96 Rue Didot
75014 Paris
France

F. J. Leal
Calle 99 No. 10–47
Santafe de Bogota
Colombia

A. Morell
Central Laboratory
Blood Transfusion Service
Swiss Red Cross
Wankdorfstrasse 10
CH-3000
Berne 22
Switzerland

A. C. Newland
Department of Haematology
The London Hospital Medical
  College
University of London
London E1 2AD
UK

F. Ramírez Osío
Clinica Infantil del Este
Calle Quelpa No. 503
Urb. El Marquez
Caracas
Venezuela

E. Rewald
Fundación Hematólogica
Corrientes 3550
7600 Mar del Plata
Argentina

V. Ruiz de Souza
Hôpital Broussais
96 Rue Didot
75014 Paris
France

J. I. Santos
Hospital Infantil de Mexico
Federico Gomez
Instituto Nacional de Salud
Dr Marquez No. 162
Mexico 7, D.F.

Preface

E. Rewald

Therapeutic applications of high-dose intravenous immunoglobulin (IVIG) have multiplied in recent times. Our purpose is to evaluate carefully the immunomodulatory possibilities of IVIG infusions. It might be appropriate to make some prior statements for the better understanding of the subject:

(1) The order of our universe may be attributed to networks. A network may be defined as a system in which there is a close functional relationship between the individual components. As a consequence, any event which affects any single component will ultimately affect the system as a whole.

(2) The investigation of chaos, a new field of knowledge, is of great help. The behavior of non-linear open systems (to which all living systems belong) cannot be foreseen, even though all known mathematical formulae are applied. Though, in spite of the chaotic condition, certain structures resembling each other may arise, and it can paradoxically be said that there exists a 'determinist chaos'. The frequency and intensity of chaotic behavior depend, among others, on 'marginal conditions' whose dimensions may be minimal. In such open systems, marginal conditions are at the same time the starting point for the sequences of a certain conduct. The lack of proportion between marginal conditions and their effects can be appreciated in the already famous 'butterfly effect' postulated by the eminent American scientist, Edward Lorenz: there exists the mathematical probability that the turbulence provoked by the fluttering of

11

a butterfly in China might trigger off, weeks later, a hurricane in the Caribbean Islands.

(3) Living systems are able to produce the necessary structures for the restoration of their integrity: they are 'autopoietic'. In consequence, they are oriented towards the maintenance of their life and the recovery of their health.

Our organism – interdependent with the environment – maintains its identity through the immunological system which is able to react with countless different antigenic determinants. The immunoglobulins are an important component of the network that makes up this system. Despite the incredible variation of stimuli to which we are exposed, the serum levels of immunoglobulins of the healthy population as a whole are remarkably similar, and this is accepted as the normal range. It is difficult to imagine that this is the result of such a diversity of idiotypes and lymphocytic clones.

By infusing high doses of IVIG, we abruptly modify the equilibrium. Marginal conditions are changed by this complex collection of molecules. That may, or may not be of benefit for the patient or may even worsen his condition. There is no doubt that it is a therapeutic resource of extreme complexity. As far as immunomodulation is concerned, it can be immediate and brief, sometimes delayed, and occasionally permanent. As will be discussed later, various mechanisms have been disclosed. In our initial studies in 1964, using massive doses of IVIG we chose as a model an attempt to prevent intrauterine death of the Rh-incompatible offspring in the sensitized mother. This scheme was self-limited by birth. Our initiative was then inspired by the hypothesis that massive infusions of immunoglobulin might induce a negative feedback response of the immunoglobulin synthesis regulation. It is noteworthy that we used similar doses to those now considered standard. The results were encouraging. At that time, only pooled IgG globulin for intramuscular use was available. We managed to administer it very carefully by the intravenous route. In one case, an anaphylactic-like reaction appeared, possibly due to the anticomplementary activity depending on the aggregation of molecules during the manufacturing process. The symptoms could be avoided when the standard commercial lyophilized IgG was diluted in fresh ACD-plasma instead of saline, and thus it was possible to increase the rate of infusions and to inject above 10 g IgG daily.

International attention was focused on the possibility of immunomodulation by high-dose IVIG when it became available for intravenous use. Besides the expected replacement therapy, Imbach and colleagues reported in 1980 a striking recovery of the platelet count in a case of autoimmune thrombocytopenic purpura. That was the starting point of the popularity of immunomodulation using IVIG.

In conclusion, you may be aware that immunomodulation by high-dose IVIG obtained from thousands of apparently healthy donors is a therapeutic resource of immense complexity, which may influence in one way or another, a broad spectrum of disease states. Much work has already been done, but much more is expected to be performed in the future.

1

Lucky strikes and mishaps in the development and clinical use of human immunoglobulins

A. Hässig

During World War II, Edwin J. Cohn[1] and his group in Boston developed the alcohol fractionation techniques subsequently named after him, for human blood plasma. The purpose of these efforts was to provide the US Navy with albumin solutions suitable for the primary resuscitation of patients with hemorrhagic shock and severe burns. The US Army used pooled lyophilized blood plasma in such cases. This fractionation yielded, as a by-product, the hemostatically active fraction I and γ-globulin: this was a first lucky strike. Cohn demanded that clinicians test on themselves whether these preparations were free of side-effects, and in this context, Janeway[2] experienced untoward effects when using γ-globulin intravenously. For this reason it was decided to restrict its administration to the intramuscular route. In retrospect, we deal here with an obvious mishap: this procedure deviated from a basic principle of transfusion therapy, which consists in substituting missing blood cells and plasma components until they approach or reach normal values. In fact, the intramuscular injection of some milliliters of a 16% γ-globulin solution adds only a few percent to the total circulation pool. Thus, the usage of γ-globulins, if we disregard immunodeficiency syndromes, was limited to the seroprophylaxis of measles and hepatitis. This was a mishap because the 'dose finding' for additional indications started with low doses that were increased only gradually. This situation persisted until 1980, when Imbach and colleagues[3], with astounding success, chose physiological and supraphysiological doses for the treatment of patients suffering from idiopathic thrombocytopenic purpura (ITP). These doses are still considered as being high!

In Switzerland, the history of the clinical use of immunoglobulins developed as follows[4]: when the US forces left Europe in 1945, the Swiss health authorities received from the Americans 13 413 units of dried plasma that were distributed by the Swiss Red Cross (SRC) among various hospitals. This generous gift was instrumental in the decision of the SRC, on 8 May 1947, to transform their Army Blood Donation Organization, established during the years of World War II, into a civil institution and to create in Berne a central laboratory with the purpose of producing dried human blood plasma suitable for clinical use. As this project materialized, it soon became evident that the pooled plasma, obtained from 30–70 donations, was heavily contaminated with hepatitis viruses. It was therefore mandatory to reduce, via the preparation of single-donor dried plasma, the frequency with which hepatitis was transmitted via blood products to that observed with single whole-blood transfusions. The relatively high content of some of the plasma units in anti-A and anti-B alloantibodies was an obstacle to the general use of these products, irrespective of the receiver's blood group. Therefore, from the early 1950s onwards, we have emphatically supported the plasma fractionation studies led by Nitschmann in Berne.

The results of these efforts comprise the first pasteurizable plasma protein solution and the first lyophilized small pool fraction I according to Cohn. Furthermore, we possessed the γ-globulin preparations for intramuscular application, and during the same period, the 1950s, Barandun and Cottier and colleagues[5] carried out their studies on immunodeficiency syndromes, especially those of a humoral nature. In the course of this work, Barandun and colleagues[6,7] identified anticomplementary IgG aggregates as the main cause of the untoward side-effects observed after intravenous administration of Cohn's γ-globulin concentrate. Based on these findings, Schultze and Schwick[8] from the Behringwerke in Marburg, Germany, decided to partially digest γ-globulin by the use of pepsin, analogous to the 'purification' of antitoxic horse serum. As in the case of animal sera thus modified, the antibody activity of pepsin-treated γ-globulin remained intact. The first γ-globulin suitable for intravenous administration, i.e. without untoward side-effects was thus developed (Gammavenin®, Behring).

16

Our intentions were to preserve the nature of intravenous immuno-globulin (IVIG) as far as possible. In this context, the chance observation that acidification was sufficient to eliminate the anticomplementarity of intramuscular immunoglobulin[9], led to the development of the pH 4 γ-globulin SRC, the forerunner of Sandoglobulin® (Sandoz). This was a lucky strike because, for the first time, we had a preparation at hand that exhibited the intact functions of the entire γ-globulin molecule, i.e. not only epitope recognition but also effector functions, in particular Fc receptor binding and complement activation.

For many years, chemically modified γ-globulins dominated the world market. The idea behind the development of such preparations was to deprive the molecules of their complement-activating capacity when they specifically bind to epitopes. This approach proved to be a memorable mishap, because these preparations, arrived at by treatment with β-propiolactone, sulfitolysis or reduction and alkylation, are, like enzymatically split γ-globulins, able to detoxify certain exotoxins (e.g. tetanus toxin) by virtue of their antibody specificity. They are not, however, suited to achieve optimal opsonophagocytosis – the hallmark of antimicrobial defense – because to attain this goal they should possess intact Fc- and C3b-binding structures: it is well known that antigen-antibody complexes in the form of Fc–C3b heterodimers are the most potent opsonizers for phagocytes. Therefore, it comes as no surprise that chemically modified γ-globulin preparations are functionally much inferior to those, such as Sandoglobulin® (Sandoz), that are basically intact molecules, and from which IgG aggregates have been selectively removed. Furthermore, the *in vivo* half-life of chemically altered γ-globulins is markedly shortened. We therefore suggest that registration authorities should withdraw such obsolete products from the market. In 1960, for an IVIG preparation to be accepted, it was sufficient that it had retained its epitope recognition capacity and that it was free from anticomplement aggregates.

By contrast, in 1982 the World Health Organization formulated the following minimum requirements for IVIG preparations[10]:

(1) Intact molecules with normal recognition activity of the Fab portion and normal effector functions on the Fc portion;

(2) Normal subclass distribution;

(3)   Normal half-life in circulation;

(4)   No unwanted side-effects *in vivo*; and

(5)   No transmission of viral diseases (hepatitis, AIDS etc.).

As already mentioned, in 1980 Imbach and co-workers[3], at the Pediatric Clinic, University of Berne, made the epochal observation that IVIG infusion in amounts corresponding to the total mass of circulating IgG produced a dramatic rise in the platelet count of patients with ITP, and thus stopped the bleeding tendency. This important finding opened the way for the concept of immunomodulation of the mononuclear phagocyte system by immunoglobulins, that is supposedly independent of their antibody specificity. Based on observations made by Fehr, i.e. that this type of IVIG treatment slows down the clearance of anti-D-loaded erythrocytes, this was termed 'reticuloendothelial system (RES) blockade'.

In 1984, Sultan and colleagues[11] reported on the successful treatment of hemophiliacs deficient in factor VIII and exhibiting autoimmune responses against this factor. They thus initiated the concept of anti-idiotypic suppression of autoimmune reactions by IVIG.

Both these discoveries were lucky strikes, as they expanded the spectrum of IVIG applicability beyond its original use as an IgG substitute in patients with hypo- or agammaglobulinemia.

We theorize today that observations made in relation to endotoxin effects *in vivo* might well shed further light on the mechanisms involved in IVIG therapy. Endotoxins of gram-negative bacteria are potent stimulators of mononuclear phagocytes, causing macrophages to release proinflammatory cytokines such as interleukin-1 (IL-1), tumor necrosis factor (TNF), and IL-6. These activate, among others, the neuroendocrine hypothalamic–pituitary–adrenal axis, thus enhancing the release and activity of glucocorticosteroids[12]. This type of stress response, in conjunction with other mechanisms such as paracrine interactions between macrophages and lymphoplasmocellular elements, participates in the suppression of specific immunoactivity.[13]

For many years, attempts have been made to abrogate the induced toxic effects of endotoxins, initially by the use of polyclonal and then monoclonal antibodies directed against the core region, including lipid A, of this bacterial lipopolysaccharide. So far, these intensive efforts have not led to a convincing success. It is against this background that earlier observations made by Iwata and colleagues[14] of the Sankyo Company in Tokyo, deserve renewed interest. They showed, both in animal experiments and in cell cultures, that intact IgG preparations are able to hinder or suppress the production and release of proinflammatory cytokines. These findings were recently extended by the observation that IVIG administration is apt to induce the formation and release of IL-1 receptor antagonists[15]. As it is more and more recognized that endotoxins act not primarily via direct toxicity, but indirectly, i.e. via an excessive release of proinflammatory mediators, especially monokines, this work should be given particular attention: it supports the notion that intact IgG exerts a dampening effect on the exocytotic activity of cells, particularly those of the mononuclear phagocyte system. This mechanism may in part be responsible for the beneficial and even, to some extent, life-saving effects obtained by Dominioni and associates[16] in treating 'septic' patients with relatively high doses of IVIG. There is also little doubt that the onset of an adult respiratory distress syndrome in which the activation of pulmonary macrophages and the consecutive release of cytokines seem to play a prominent role, can be delayed or even prevented by high-dose IVIG therapy. The latter is also effective when given preoperatively, in reducing infection and mortality in patients at risk for sepsis undergoing sugery for colorectal cancer[17]. A recently published monograph[18] on gut-derived infectious–toxic shock is in line with these thoughts. It is proposed that this subtype of septic shock, in which splanchnic ischemia, reperfusion damage of the gut wall, consecutive intestinal barrier failure, a multispecies bacterial attack and a progressive inflammatory cascade appear to be in the foreground of pathogenctic mechanisms, may be especially amenable to high-dose IVIG prophylaxis. It is expected that in such cases early and high-dose IVIG administration is apt to involve the following beneficial actions:

(1) Improved opsonophagocytosis, especially by neutrophils, where it should be remembered that 70–80% of antimicrobial specificities of circulating IgGs are directed against the surface epitopes of intestinal bacteria;

(2) Down-regulation of the release of inflammatory mediators from cells, especially mononuclear phagocytes, and up-regulation of monokine receptor antagonist release; and

(3) Restitution of more harmonious neuroendocrine functions, with up-regulation of specific immunofunctions.

There is good reason to assume that IVIG preparations with intact Fab and Fc functions will, in the future, play a central role in reducing the mortality of surgical patients in intensive care.

Another problem concerns idiotype–anti-idiotype interactions and their relationship to neuroendocrine mechanisms of immunosuppression. The phenomenon of oligoclonality in autoimmune disorders might well be due to an immunoendocrine imbalance, in which a moderately elevated blood level of free bioactive cortisol favors the transition of immunoglobulin polyclonality to relative oligoclonality with a tendency towards autoimmune reactions. One can speculate that a further increase in the blood level of free cortisol may lead to a 'freeze' of specific immune responses, i.e. a total incapacity of the organism to mount specific primary immune reactions, and a marked reduction of its ability to carry out recall responses; if this process develops further, opportunistic microorganisms are apt to attain clinical relevance and the organism becomes an easy prey for nosocomial microbes. In this context, the cortisol-sparing effect of IVIG therapy in patients with otherwise glucocorticoid-dependent autoimmune diseases and asthma, as shown by Gelfand and Mazer[19], deserves our particular attention. There are certain parallels between this phenomenon and the effect of glycosaminoglycans (GAGs) in patients with iatrogenic Cushing's syndrome[20,21]. In fact, immunoglobulins and GAGs predominate in the restitutive phase following systemic sequelae of inflammation, whereas the acute phase of the latter is characterized by a leading role of proinflammatory mediators (e.g. monokines) and glucocorticoids. In constrast to these, which are non-curative inhibitors of inflammation, IVIG may exert a truly curative action.

Thus, 50 years after Cohn's pioneering work, we are left with still more to do!

ACKNOWLEDGEMENTS

The studies on gammaglobulins carried out in Berne were the result of teamwork to which Silvio Barandun, Hans Cottier, Hans Friedli, Andreas Gardi, Paul Imbach, Henri Isliker, Peter Kistler, Andreas

Morell and Urs Nydegger made major contributions. The success of Sandoglobulin® (Sandoz) was initiated by Max Täschler, Charles Studer of Sandoz Basel, Hans Bühlmann, Konradin Knöpfel of Sandoz Nürnberg and its producer, the Central Laboratory of the Swiss Red Cross Blood Transfusion Service, Berne.

REFERENCES

1. Cohn, E. J. (1948). The history of plasma fractionation. In Andrus, E. C., Bronk, D. W., Carden, G. A., Keefer, C. S., Lockwood, J. S., Wearn, J. T. and Winternitz, M. C. (eds.) *Advances in Military Medicine*, Vol. 1, pp. 364–443. (Boston:Little Brown)
2. Janeway, C. A. (1970). The development of clinical uses of immuno-globulins: A review. In Merler, E. (ed.) *Immunoglobulins, Biologic Aspects and Clinical Uses*, pp. 3–14. (Washington:National Academy of Sciences)
3. Imbach, P. S., Barandun, S., d'Apuzzo, V., Baumgartner, C., Hirt, A., Morell, A., Rossi, E., Vest, M. and Wagner, H. P. (1980). High dose intravenous gammaglobulin for idiopathic thrombocytopenic purpura in childhood. *Lancet*, **1**, 1228
4. Hässig, A. (1991). 50 Jahre Blutspendedienst des Schweizerischen Roten Kreuzes. *Schweiz. Med. Wschr.*, **121**, 156
5. Barandun, S., Cottier, H., Hässig, A. and Riva, G. (1959). *Das Antikörper-mangelsyndrom.* Benno Schwabe & Co. Basel/Stuttgart; Sonderdruck aus der *Helv. Med. Acta*, **26**, 111–539
6. Barandun, S., Kistler, P., Jeunet, F. and Isliker, H. (1962). Intravenous administration of human γ-globulin. *Vox Sang.*, **7**, 158
7. Barandun, S. (1964). *Die Gammaglobulin-Therapie. Chemische, Immunologische und Klinische Grundlagen*, Vol. 17. (Basel:Bibl. Haematol.)
8. Schultze, H. E. and Schwick, G. (1962). Ueber neue Möglichkeiten intravenöser Gammaglobulin-Applikation. *Dtsch. Med. Wschr.*, **87**, 1643
9. Hässig, A. (1991). One hundred years of passive immunization: from anti-toxic animal sera to human γ-globulins. *Sandorama*, **3**, 19–21
10. WHO Expert Committee on Biological Standardization (1982). *Report of an Informal Meeting on Intravenous Immunoglobulins (Human)*. Geneva, November 29–December 1
11. Sultan, Y., Kazatchkine, M. D., Maisonneuve, P. and Nydegger, U. E. (1984). Antiidiotypic suppression of auto-antibodies to factor VIII anti-hemophilic factor by high-dose intravenous gammaglobulin. *Lancet*, **1**, 765

12. Besedovsky, H. O. and del Rey, A. (1991). Physiological implication of the immune neuroendocrine network. In Ader, R., Felten, D. L. and Cohen, N. (eds.) *Psychoneuroimmunology*, 2nd edn. (New York:Academic Press)
13. Intravenous Immunoglobulin Collaborative Study Group (1992). Prophylactic intravenous administration of standard immune globulin as compared with core-lipopolysaccharide immunoglobulin in patients at high risk of postsurgical infection. *N. Engl. J. Med.*, **327**, 234
14. Iwata, M., Shimozato, R., Tokiwa, H. and Tsubura, E. (1986). Antipyretic activity of human immunoglobulin preparations for intravenous use in an experimental model of fever in rabbits. In Morell, A. and Nydegger, U. E. (eds.) *Clinical Use of Intravenous Immunoglobulins*, p. 327. (London:Academic Press)
15. Fischer, E., Van Zee, K. J., Marano, M. A., Rock, C. S., Kenney, J. S., Poutsiaka, D. D., Dinarello, Ch. A., Lowry, S. F. and Moldawer, L. L. (1992). Interleukin-1 receptor antagonist circulates in experimental inflammation and in human disease. *Blood*, **79**, 2196
16. Dominioni, L., Dionigi, R., Fanello, M., Chiaranda, M., Acquatolo, A., Ballabio, A. and Sguotti, C. (1992). Effects of high dose IgG on survival of surgical patients with sepsis scores of 20 or greater. *Arch. Surg.*, **126**, 236
17. Cafiero, F., Gipponi, M., Bonalumi, U., Piccardo, A., Sguotti, Ch. and Corbetta, G. (1992). Prophylaxis of infection with intravenous immunoglobulins plus antibiotic for patients at risk for sepsis undergoing surgery for colorectal cancer: result of a randomized multicenter clinical trial. *Surgery*, **112**, 24
18. Cottier, H. and Kraft, R. (eds.) (1992). Gut-Derived Infectious-Toxic Shock (GITS). *Current Studies in Hematology and Blood Transfusion*, No. 59. (Basel: Karger)
19. Gelfand, E. W. and Mazer, B. D. (1993). Intravenous γ-globulin: an alternative treatment in severe steroid-dependent asthma. In Rewald, E. and Morrell, A. (eds.) *Immunomodulation by Intravenous Immunoglobulin*. (Casterton UK:Parthenon Publishing)
20. Annefeld, M. (1989). Der dosisabhängige Effekt von Glykosaminglukan-Peptid Komplex auf den durch Koritikosteroide gestörten Stoffwechsel im Knorpelgewebe von Ratten. *Z. Rheumatol.*, **48**, 188
21. Stellon, A., Davies, A., Wegg, A. and Williams, R. (1986). Microcrystalline hydroxyapatite compound in prevention of bone loss in corticosteroid-treated patients with chronic hepatitis. *Postgrad. Med. J.*, **61**, 791

2

Gut-derived infectious–toxic shock

H. Cottier and R. Kraft

The optimal management of septic shock following major surgery, severe burns and other severe trauma remains one of the major unresolved problems in surgery and medicine. Despite great progress in supportive care and antibiotic therapy, the fatality rate of these conditions remains high[1]. Continuation of the search into novel prophylactic and therapeutic strategies in this field is thus urgently needed[2].

Often, but by no means always, bacteremia accompanies septic shock, and gram-negative microorganisms predominate among the isolates[3]. This points to the gut as a major source of infection in these conditions. Sepsis in the original sense, i.e. progressive hematogeneous propagation and generalization of infection, does not seem to be a prerequisite for shock, adult respiratory distress syndrome (ARDS) and multiple organ failure (MOF) to occur in this context. Rather, an excessive uncontrolled escalation of proinflammatory cascades with toxic effects appears to be the pathogenetic hallmark[4]. If the invasion of bacteria commences in the intestinal tract, be it local or – as happens quite frequently – more diffuse, we speak of gut-derived infectious–toxic shock (GITS), an important subtype of septic shock. Recent findings have contributed to a more profound insight into the mechanisms involved. Since a rational and efficient prophylaxis and therapy depends on our knowledge of the pathogenesis of this particular disorder, we shall briefly consider some important aspects of the origin and progression of GITS.

THE INTESTINAL BARRIER AND ITS FAILURE

The mutualistic relationship among the hundreds of enteric microbial species, and between the intestinal microflora and the host, is the result of an evolutionary process of long duration. Under physiological conditions, the macroorganism benefits from the presence of this mass of microorganisms in many ways, and specialized bacteria form and maintain a 'protective colonization' on the inner surface of the digestive tract[5]. In the healthy adult, the mass of intestinal microorganisms is contained within the lumen by an intricate system of structural and functional obstacles[6]. In brief, this comprises, from inside to outside, secretory IgA and lysozyme, which are in part associated with mucus[7]; the enterocyte layer, covered by the glycocalyx, tightened by the intercellular junctional complex, particularly the zonulae occludentes, and equipped with protective molecules such as interferon and enzymes; and the mucosal stroma which harbors, for example, antibodies, complement, granulocytes, macrophages, lymphocytes, plasma cells and natural killer cells as well as lymphatics and small blood vessels (Figure 1). Lymphoid follicles in the intestinal wall function primarily as immunological contact

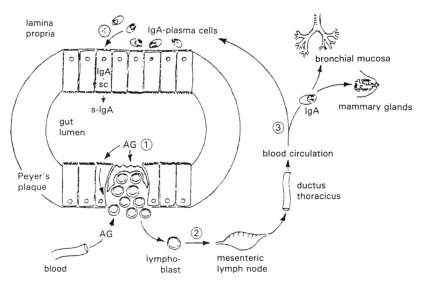

Figure 1 Schematic representation of the intestinal wall and the gut-associated lymphoid tissue. AG, antigen. Reproduced with kind permission from reference 6

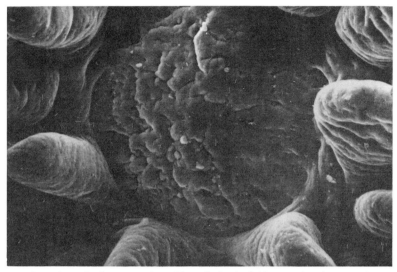

Figure 2 Peyer's patch of a mouse, viewed from the luminal side (scanning electron micrograph)

structures, in as much as they are covered by a specialized epithelium with so-called 'M' cells that are permeable for macromolecules, e.g. antigens and small particles (Figure 2)[8]. Taken together, the various components of the intestinal barrier provide for both a tight seclusion of, and a constant but restricted contact of the host with, the intestinal microflora and/or intraluminal antigens. The integrity of the intestinal barrier, in particular that of the epithelial layer, depends on a sufficient supply of oxygen and nutrients[9], and especially of arginine and glutamine[10].

Intestinal barrier failure can occur in various ways. Trivial causes are, for instance, physical disruption, acute ulceration/perforation, and suture insufficiencies in the gut wall. More complex damaging mechanisms include severe disturbances of the ecological balance in the intestinal microflora, and endotoxin effects. Cytotoxic chemicals and ionizing radiation represent well-established noxious agents that attack, among other, the intestinal epithelium. However, particularly important causes are splanchnic ischemia[11] and consecutive reperfusion damage, involving oxygen-derived radicals[12]. The lesions produced by this type of injury may range from a break-up of tight junctions[13] to epithelial necrosis and mucosal denudation (Figure 3). Of importance in the present context is the fact that regeneration of the enterocyte layer after subtotal destruction requires 4 or more days[14].

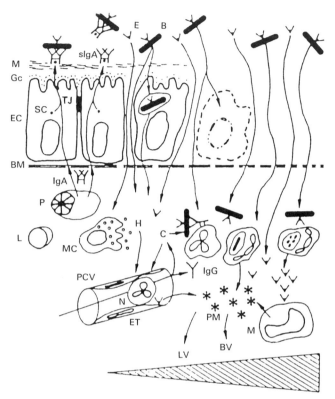

Figure 3 Simplified scheme of events following a disruption of the intestinal barrier due to ischemia and reperfusion damage, with early bacterial attack, influx of endotoxin, and inflammatory reaction. From left to right, normal mucosa to increasing barrier damage. B, gram-negative bacterium; E, endotoxin; M, mucus; Gc, glycocalyx; EC, enterocyte; TJ, tight junction; BM, basement membrane; P, plasma cell; IgA, dimeric immunoglobulin A, linked to J chain; SC, secretory component; sIgA, secretory IgA; IgG, immunoglobulin G antibodies; L, lymphocyte; MC, mast cell; H, histamine; PCV, postcapillary venule; N, neutrophil; C, complement; M, macrophage; PM, proinflammatory mediators; LV, lymph vessel; BV, small blood vessel. Reproduced with kind permission from reference 4

ASSUMED AND PROVEN IMMEDIATE CONSEQUENCES OF ACUTE INTESTINAL BARRIER FAILURE

Markedly increased bacterial translocation from the gut lumen into the intestinal wall, to regional lymph nodes and even into the general circulation, is a well-documented consequence of a partial or complete

Table 1 Stages in bacterial translocation pathogenesis

Promoting mechanism	Mesenteric lymph node	Spleen	Liver	Blood	Death
(1) Mucosal barrier disruption	1st stage →				
(2) Intestinal bacterial overgrowth	1st stage →				
(3) Immunocompromised host		2nd stage →			
Non-lethal combination			3rd stage →		
Lethal combination			3rd stage		→

Modified from reference 15

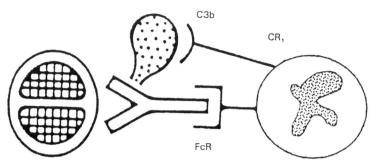

Figure 4 Immune opsonophagocytosis at a bacterium (left, enlarged): attachment of the microbe to a neutrophil (right) with the help of both specific antibody and complement. FcR, receptor for the Fc portion of immunoglobulins (mainly IgG); CR_1, receptor for the C3b fragment of the third component of complement. Modified, with kind permission from reference 52

breakdown of the enterocyte layer integrity[15] (Table 1). In view of the innumerable microbial species present in the distal digestive tract, it can be assumed that an acute intestinal barrier failure opens the way for a multibacterial attack[4]. Success or failure of antimicrobial defense is often decided in the early phase of infection[16]. Neutrophils, in conjunction

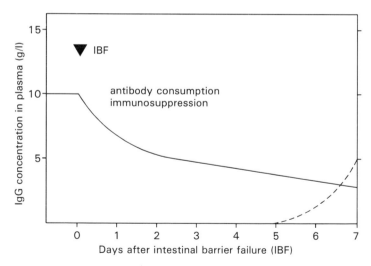

Figure 5 IgG concentration in the circulating blood as a function of time after intestinal barrier failure (IBF). The dashed line represents the host's own humoral immune response

with specific antibodies, are especially suited for rapidly combating the invaders, and C3b–IgG heterodimers have been shown to be particularly effective opsonizers for microorganisms (Figure 4)[17]. This observation, and the high probability that we deal here with a multispecies bacterial challenge, suggest that antibodies, also those of the IgG class, will be consumed rapidly in such a process. It has in fact been reported that the level of circulating IgG may fall in the course of septic shock, to about 50% of normal (Figure 5)[18]. This situation may be likened to a transient antibody deficiency, and will be discussed later. The further course of events following acute intestinal barrier disruption largely depends on the outcome of antimicrobial defense in the early phase of the process.

INFLAMMATORY REACTION: BENEFITS AND HAZARDS

In most instances, the complex inflammatory reaction fulfils its protective functions in as much as it succeeds, with the help of specific immune responses, in overcoming invading microbes and/or in restoring tissue integrity[19]. In the case of intestinal barrier failure, regeneration of the intestinal layer is a prerequisite for the phlogistic reaction to calm down.

If, however, the aggressive agents – microorganisms and/or toxins – continue or even enhance their attack, inflammation may progressively build up and reach a level where it gets out of antagonistic control. In such a situation, the powerful forces of defense are apt to direct themselves against the host and put his or her life in acute danger, mainly via the action of proinflammatory mediators. Apart from the complement, coagulation and kinin systems, certain cytokines, especially tumor necrosis factor (TNF)[20], interferon-γ (IFN-γ)[21], interleukin-1 (IL-1)[22], and others, play a dominant role and in part interact among each other. Additional mediators, such as platelet-activating factor (PAF)[23], certain eicosanoids[24], oxygen-derived radicals[25], proteinases liberated by phagocytes[26], and others, participate in this deleterious cascade (Figure 6). The plasma levels of elastase-α_1-protease inhibitor (E-α_1 PI) complex, neopterin, endotoxin and TNF yield some information on the development and outcome of GITS[27]. The onset of an ARDS may signal a developing MOF.

29

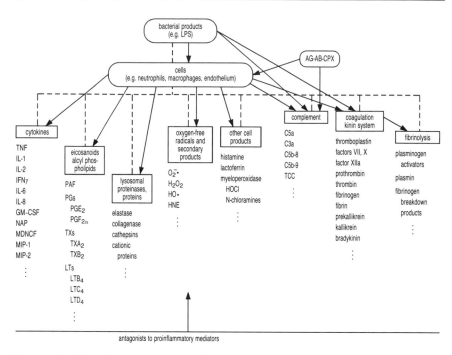

Figure 6 Schematic representation of proinflammatory mediator cascades elicited by endotoxin (LPS) and other bacterial products. Arrows indicate activation; dashed lines indicate synergistic and/or sequential relationships between groups of factors, including positive and, less frequently, negative feedback loops; AG–AB–CPX, antigen–antibody complexes; TNF, tumor necrosis factor; IL, interleukin; IFN, interferon; GM-CSF, granulocyte–monocyte colony stimulating factor; PAF, platelet-activating factor; PG, prostaglandin; TX, thromboxane; LT, leukotriene

ROLE OF BACTERIAL ENDOTOXIN

In the case of infection by gram-negative bacteria, endotoxin, a lipo-polysaccharide (LPS) constituent of the outer microbial membrane seems to play a leading role in triggering the excessive proinflammatory reaction mentioned above. Although a direct toxicity of LPS is difficult to demonstrate, its markedly stimulating effect on a variety of cell types, especially macrophages, has been well documented[28]. Thus, endotoxin (and in particular its toxic lipid A component, which is normally hidden by the outer constituents of the bacterial membrane) threatens the integrity of the macroorganism as soon as it is freed in greater amounts

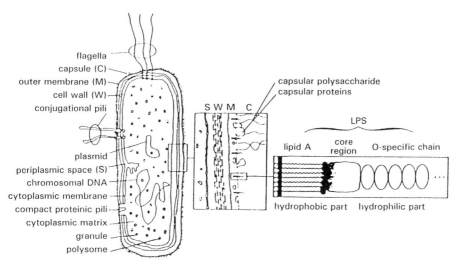

Figure 7 Schematic illustration of the ultrastructural and macromolecular composition of a gram–negative bacterium. LPS is the chemical designation for endotoxin, which is an integral part of the microbial outer membrane. Reproduced with kind permission from Lebek, G. and Cottier, H. (1992). Notes on the bacterial content of the gut. In Cottier, H. and Kraft, R. (eds.) *Gut-Derived Infectious–Toxic Shock (GITS). Current Studies in Hematology and Blood Transfusion*, No. 59, pp. 1–18. (Basel:Karger)

and enters into contact with responsive cells (Figure 7). It has been proposed that, under physiological conditions, the gut mucosa is impervious and resistant to LPS[29]. However, information on the amount of free endotoxin in the intestinal lumen is scarce. Substantial release of endotoxin occurs mainly from damaged or dead gram–negative bacteria, for instance in a partially degraded, highly active form from disintegrating phagocytes that had engulfed the microbes[30]. Other mechanisms of LPS release comprise noxious effects of antibiotics on the microorganisms, and rapid proliferation of the latter.

The fate of endotoxin liberated in the tissue remains to be clarified. It may be neutralized by naturally occurring anti–LPS antibodies, although these could rapidly be consumed[31], or it may bind to LPS-binding protein (LBP), lipoproteins, antithrombin III, α_2-macroglobulin and/or other, poorly characterized plasma proteins[29]. The elimination of such endotoxin–protein complexes seems to be achieved primarily by the liver.

It should be pointed out that enhanced endotoxin release is no absolute prerequisite for septic shock to develop, since such complications occur also with severe infections due to gram-positive microorganisms[32].

31

DISTURBED IMMUNE FUNCTIONS IN
DEVELOPING SEPTIC SHOCK

In addition to consumptive antibody deficiency, as mentioned above, a developing septic shock affects the immune apparatus in many other ways. Loss of intestinal barrier integrity goes along with impaired production of secretory IgA. In addition, and probably even more importantly, major trauma, major surgery and severe burns are known to be followed by marked immunosuppression. The mechanisms responsible for this 'post-trauma-surgery-burns (TSB)' immuno-deficiency syndrome[33] are still not completely understood. They are complex and appear to involve, among others, enhanced suppressor activity of cells, lymphocyte sequestration, release of suppressor peptides, phagocyte dysfunction and hormonal effects[34].

POSSIBLE NOVEL STRATEGIES FOR PROPHYLAXIS
AND THERAPY OF GITS

Although it has been stated that 'the time has passed when the management of septic shock could be summarized as supportive care and the administration of antibiotics'[35], the future development of immuno-prophylaxis and therapy in this field is difficult to predict. Various conceptual avenues have been followed, but so far no approach has reached the stage of undisputable clinical usefulness.

Septic shock resulting in multiple organ damage has aptly been termed 'host defense failure'[36]. Since it is known to occur preferentially in individuals with age-associated debilitating disorders[37] and/or reduced nutritional status[38], it is tempting to introduce prophylactic measures wherever possible. This is mainly the case for preoperative patients with a high risk of developing infectious-toxic complications after major surgery. The best risk prognosticators appear to be age, lowered blood albumin concentration and diminished cell-mediated immunoreactivity, tested on the skin[39]. Various possibilities have been considered to improve the patient's condition in such a situation; however, there is an astounding scarcity of clinical reports dealing with non-specific prophylactic immunostimulation and/or nutritional support in these cases. Most efforts at present focus on specific passive immunization with antibodies that can primarily act as anti-infectious or antitoxic agents.

Anti-infectious passive immunization

This comprises the use of polyclonal or (less frequently) monoclonal antibodies directed against O-, K-, H- and/or other antigens of gram-negative bacteria, which predominate in the causation of GITS. A large proportion, if not the bulk of antibodies in pooled, polyspecific human immunoglobulins such as Sandoglobulin® (Sandoz), especially standard IgG for intravenous use, is directed against the innumerable antigens of intestinal bacteria. This can be deduced both from titrating these preparations with a multitude of enteric microorganisms[40] and from the fact that, in small rodents[41] as well as in humans[42], the lymph nodes draining the gut undergo a postnatal antigen-driven expansion which by far exceeds the one seen in lymph nodes in other locations.

In view of the immediate multispecies bacterial attack associated with acute intestinal barrier failure, the early administration of intravenous immunoglobulin (IVIG) seems indicated after such an event. Theoretically, it should be given until the enteric epithelial layer is regenerated and the barrier is thus restored. This may last a week or more. The notion that prophylactic, or at least early, passive immunization with IVIG has a good chance of improving the patient's condition, finds

Table 2 Prophylactic use of intravenous immunoglobulins (IVIG) in patients at risk of developing septic shock

Authors	Dose of IVIG (g/kg body weight)	Major beneficial effect	Significance
Duswald *et al.* (1980)[43]	0.25*	reduced frequency of postoperative local infections	+
Cafiero and Gipponi (1989)[18]	0.2* (+ postoperative days 1 and 5)	reduced lethality	+
IVIG Collaborative Study Group (1992)[16]	0.4 (+ postoperative days 7 and 14)	reduced incidence of local infections and pulmonary complications	+

*, Approximate values

33

considerable support in clinical observations made so far. In 1980, Duswald and colleagues[43] gave 20 g of IVIG to patients shortly before major surgery (Table 2). The treated group suffered significantly fewer postoperative infectious complications as compared to controls. Analogous observations, including a reduction in the frequency of pulmonary complications, were subsequently made by other authors[18,44]. Of even greater importance is that IVIG has a protective action when given early after severe injury. Glinz and co-workers[45] treated polytraumatized individuals with 12 g IVIG per person on admission to hospital, as well as 5 and 12 days later. Despite these rather low doses of pooled IgG, the patients experienced significantly fewer pulmonary complications than did the controls. The incidence of late sepsis in this series was, however, not significantly different between the two groups. A clearly measurable improvement of condition was noticed in intensive care patients given modest doses of IVIG, enriched with some IgM and IgA, on admission and 12, 24 and 36 h later[46]. Somewhat similar doses of IVIG, i.e. 0.4 g/kg body weight, given 1 day after admission to the intensive care unit, plus 0.2 g/kg thereafter and 'when needed', another 0.4 g/kg after 5 days, led to a shortening of the fever period, a drop in the numbers of positive blood cultures from 40% to 8%, and a reduction in the need for antibiotics from 95% to 38%. The lethality in the group of IVIG-treated patients was 58%, as compared to 75% in the controls[47]. Even better results were obtained by Dominioni and colleagues[48], who treated surgical patients with a sepsis score of 20 and greater with 0.4 g/kg of IVIG on admission, repeated 1 and 5 days later: the lethality in the IVIG-supplemented group was 38% and that in the control group 67%. The impression is thus gained that high doses of IVIG, and not only early administration, are of paramount importance for this type of treatment to be successful. In fact, it has been reported that patients in whom the concentration of IgG in the blood plasma was kept above 10 g/l by supplementation with IVIG, rarely developed postoperative infectious complications[18]. The observations made by the Italian authors[48] compare favorably with the results obtained with IVIG treatment in severely burned patients[49], for whom this type of therapy is widely accepted. The hesitation to use IVIG more broadly in critical situations such as developing septic shock most probably stems from the fact that these preparations are rather expensive. However, solid cost–benefit comparisons in this field are lacking. We should consider in this context that, in contrast for example, to progressive cancer, we deal here with a short-lasting, transient life-threatening crisis, where survival is usually synonymous with regaining health. The shortened stay in the intensive care unit should also be included in the cost–benefit calculations.

There is no convincing evidence that pooled human IgG contains protective anticore LPS antibodies[50]. It seems reasonable, therefore, to assume that the beneficial effects of IVIG above-mentioned rely primarily on the presence, in these preparations, of protective antibodies directed against serotype-specific antigens on gram-negative and other bacteria that participate in the multispecies microbial attack following intestinal barrier failure. The pre-existing pool of these antibodies is apt to be consumed rapidly in the course of such an event. In line with this notion is the fact that the level of circulating IgG exhibits a rapid fall early after major surgery in the 'at-risk' patient, and that this phenomenon can be corrected by the administration of IVIG, concomitant with a reduction in the number of postoperative infectious episodes[51].

In addition to its anti-infectious action – mainly via enhancing immunophagocytosis of microbes, i.e. mostly neutrophils[52] – IVIG may also exert a beneficial immunomodulatory effect, for example by dampening inflammatory reactions[53].

So-called 'hyperimmune' IVIG preparations with high titers of antibodies directed against particular bacterial serotypes, e.g. 'Pseudomonas-Igs', have been used with considerable success in patients with *Pseudomonas* sepsis and septic shock[54]. The same pertains to 'hyperimmune' immunoglobulin obtained from volunteers vaccinated with a cocktail of the most frequent *Klebsiella* and *Pseudomonas* antigens[55]. This approach is apt to be especially appropriate when one or a few bacterial species have taken the lead in the infectious process.

Peroral/intraintestinal administration of pooled human immunoglobulins, either as such or in combination with IVIG, has been shown to be beneficial in patients undergoing allogeneic bone marrow transplantation[56]. To our knowledge, however, this possibility has not yet been tested on a broader scale in GITS or other forms of septic shock.

Antitoxic passive immunization

The antitoxic passive immunization of animals and/or humans before or during developing septic shock has so far been examined in two

Table 3 Possibilities of immune prophylaxis/immunotherapy in patients at risk of developing gut-derived infectious-toxic shock

Phase, leading process	Indicative symptoms/signs	Possible immunoprophylaxis therapy	Reported beneficial effects in humans	References
Preoperative prophylactic	reduced cell-mediated immune reactivity ('anergy' in skin test) risk of developing gram-negative infection	non-specific immunostimulation?	unknown	63
		vaccination against several important O-, K- and/or H-antigens of gram-negative bacteria	yes	55
Intestinal barrier failure	hemorrhagic shock splanchnic hypoperfusion	polyspecific immunoglobulins?	yes	43, 45, 47, 48, 51
Infectious toxic process	endotoxemia, commencing ARDS	anti-core LPS antibodies?	yes	58, 60
	elevated blood levels of, for example, elastase and neopterin	monoclonal antibodies directed against cytokines and/or their receptors on cells?	?	59
Severe infection especially by certain gram-negative bacteria	bacteremia, sepsis, caused by one or a few gram-negative microbial species/strains	hyperimmune immuno-globulins, possibly monoclonal antibodies against particular microbial species/strains	yes	54, 55

ARDS, adult respiratory distress syndrome; LPS, lipopolysaccharide. Modified with kind permission from reference 63 directions: on the one hand by the use of polyclonal[57] or monoclonal[58] 'anticore LPS antibodies', and on the other hand by the application of monoclonal antibodies directed against proinflammatory mediators, e.g. TNF-α[59] or IFN-γ[21]. Clinical trials centered on the effects of these two types of antitoxic passive immunization have led to inconsistent results. These have been discussed in detail[35] and will not be considered at any length here. For instance, the use of the monoclonal, supposedly 'anticore LPS' antibody HA-IA was reported to be beneficial for patients with clinically diagnosed sepsis and gram-negative bacteremia, especially for those in shock on entry into the study[60]. Conversely, 'core LPS hyperimmune globulin' was, in contrast to standard IVIG, unable to reduce the incidence of infections in a similar cohort of patients[61]. Doubts have also been expressed as to the true nature (antigen–antibody reaction or non-specific binding?) of the interaction between 'anticore LPS antibodies' and LPS[62]. Obviously, more studies are needed to clarify these problems.

Most clinical studies carried out so far have focused on one particular type of immunoprophylaxis or therapy in patients in or at risk of developing septic shock. Since the various approaches followed until today are apt to interfere optimally with different phases of the infectious–toxic process, a combination of the immunological measures outlined above may be envisaged in the future. Such a scheme could, for instance, encompass the following:

(1) Non-specific immunostimulation, nutritional support and vaccination against several important O-, K- and/or H-antigens of gram-negative bacteria in preoperative or other individuals at risk of developing GITS;

(2) Polyspecific (standard) IVIG at the time of intestinal barrier failure and for some time thereafter;

(3) 'Anticore LPS antibodies' or other endotoxin-binding agents in the phase of commencing, or existing, endotoxemia;

(4) Monoclonal antibodies directed against proinflammatory mediators and/or their receptors on cells in the period of progressive inflammation; and

(5) 'Hyperimmune immunoglobulin' against particular microbial species and strains, once they have been cultured from the blood[63] (Table 3).

REFERENCES

1. Veterans Administration Systemic Sepsis Cooperative Study Group (1987). Effect of high-dose glucocorticoid therapy on mortality in patients with clinical signs of systemic sepsis. *N. Engl. J. Med.*, **317**, 659–65
2. Goldsmith, M. F. (1991). Excitement over immunomodulation inundates clinical research meetings. *J. Am. Med. Assoc.*, **265**, 2768–73
3. Clowes, G. H. A. Jr (ed.) (1988). *Trauma, Sepsis, and Shock. The Physiological Basis of Therapy.* (New York:Marcel Dekker)
4. Kraft, R., Ruchti, C., Burkhardt, A. and Cottier, H. (1992). Pathogenetic principles in the development of gut-derived infectious-toxic shock (GITS) and multiple organ failure. In Cottier, H. and Kraft, R. (eds.) *Gut-Derived Infectious-Toxic Shock (GITS). Current Studies in Hematology and Blood Transfusion* No. 59, pp. 204–40. (Basel:Karger)
5. Savage, D. C. (1984). Overview of the association of microbes with epithelial surfaces. In Rusch, V. and Luckey, T. D. (eds.) *Microecology and Therapy. Proceedings of the IXth International Symposium on Intestinal Microecology*, Vol. 14, pp. 169–82. (Herborn)
6. Laissue, J. A. and Gebbers, J. O. (1992). The intestinal barrier and the gut-associated lymphoid tissue. In Cottier, H. and Kraft, R. (eds.) *Gut-Derived Infectious-Toxic Shock (GITS). Current Studies in Hematology and Blood Transfusion*, No. 59, pp. 19–43. (Basel:Karger)
7. Clamp, J. R. (1980). Gastrointestinal mucus. In Wright, R. (ed.) *Recent Advances in Gastrointestinal Pathology*, pp. 47–58. (London:Saunders)
8. Owen, R. L. (1977). Sequential uptake of horseradish peroxidase by lymphoid follicle epithelium of Peyer's patches in the normal unobstructed mouse intestine. *Gastroenterology*, **72**, 440–51
9. Page, C. P. (1989). The surgeon and gut maintenance. *Am. J. Surg.*, **158**, 485–90
10. Souba, W. W., Klimberg, V. S., Hautamaki, R. D., Mendenhall, W. H., Bova, F. C., Howard, R. J., Bland, K. I. and Copeland, E. M. (1990). Oral glutamine reduces bacterial translocation following abdominal radiation. *J. Surg. Res.*, **48**, 1–5
11. Fiddian-Green, R. G. (1988). Splanchnic ischaemia and multiple organ failure in the critically ill. *Ann. R. Coll. Surg. Engl.*, **70**, 128–34
12. Deitch, E. A., Bridges, W., Ma, L., Berg, R., Specian, R. D. and Granger, D. N. (1990). Hemorrhagic shock-induced bacterial translocation: the role of neutrophils and hydroxyl radicals. *J. Trauma*, **30**, 942–51
13. Deitch, E. A. (1990). Intestinal permeability is increased in burn patients shortly after injury. *Surgery*, **107**, 411–16

14. Bragg, L. E. and Thompson, J. S. (1989). The influence of resection on the growth of intestinal neomucosa. *J. Surg. Res.*, **46**, 306–10
15. Berg, R. D. (1992). Translocation of enteric bacteria in health and disease. In Cottier, H. and Kraft, R. (eds.) *Gut-Derived Infectious–Toxic Shock (GITS). Current Studies in Hematology and Blood Transfusion*, No. 59, pp. 44–65. (Basel:Karger)
16. Meakins, J. L. (1981). Clinical importance of host resistance to infection in surgical patients. *Adv. Surg.*, **15**, 225–55
17. Malbran, A., Frank, M. M. and Fries, L. F. (1987). Interactions of monomeric IgG bearing covalently bound C3b with polymorphonuclear leucocytes. *Immunology*, **61**, 15–20
18. Cafiero, F. and Gipponi, M. (1989). Profilassi delle infezioni in chirurgia per neoplasia dell'apparato digerente. In Rossi Ferrini, P. (ed.) *Impiego Clinico delle Immunoglobuline Endovena: Presente e Futuro*, pp. 63–8. (Milano: Edizioni Grafiche Mazzucchelli)
19. Iversen, O. H. (ed.) (1989). Cell kinetics of the inflammatory reaction. *Current Topics in Pathology*, Vol. 79, pp. 1–262. (Berlin:Springer)
20. Fong, Y. and Lowry, S. F. (1990). Tumor necrosis factor in the pathophysiology of infection and sepsis. *Clin. Immunol. Immunopathol.*, **55**, 157–70
21. Billiau, A. (1988). Not just cachectin involved in toxic shock. *Nature (London)*, **331**, 665
22. Offner, E., Philippé, J., Vogelaers, D., Colardyn, F., Baele, G., Baudrihaye, M., Vermeulen, A. and Leroux-Roels, G. (1990). Serum tumor necrosis factor levels in patients with infectious disease and septic shock. *J. Lab. Clin. Med.*, **116**, 100–5
23. Braquet, P., Touqui, L., Shen, T. Y. and Vargaftig, B. B. (1987). Perspectives in platelet-activating factor research. *Pharmacol. Rev.*, **39**, 97–145
24. Hechtman, H. B., Welbourn, R., Goldman, G., Patterson, I. S., Klausner, J. M., Valeri, C. R. and Shepro, D. (1990). Activation of neutrophils and the role of eicosanoids in the initiation of organ failure. In Schlag, G., Redl, H. and Siegel, J. H. (eds.) *Shock, Sepsis, and Organ Failure*, pp. 357–73. (Berlin:Springer)
25. Taylor, A. E., Matalon, S. and Ward, P. (eds.) (1986). *Physiology of Oxygen Radicals*. (Bethesda:American Physiological Society)
26. Neuhof, H. (1990). Role of proteinases in the pathophysiology of organ failure. In Schlag, G., Redl, H. and Siegel, J. H. (eds.) *Shock, Sepsis, and Organ Failure*, pp. 404–20. (Berlin:Springer)
27. Lundsgaard-Hansen, P. and Blauhut, B. (1992). Markers and mediators in enterogenic infectious–toxic shock. In Cottier, H. and Kraft, R. (eds.) *Gut-Derived Infectious–Toxic Shock (GITS). Current Studies in Hematology and Blood Transfusion*, No. 59, pp. 163–203. (Basel:Karger)

28. Doran, J. E. (1992). Biological effects of endotoxin. In Cottier, H. and Kraft, R. (eds.) *Gut-Derived Infectious–Toxic Shock (GITS). Current Studies in Hematology and Blood Transfusion*, No. 59, pp. 66–99. (Basel:Karger)

29. Bayston, K. F. and Cohen, J. (1990). Bacterial endotoxin and current concepts in the diagnosis and treatment of endotoxaemia. *J. Med. Microbiol.*, **31**, 73–83

30. Duncan, R. L. Jr, Hoffman, J., Tesh, V. L. and Morrison, D. C. (1986). Immunologic activity of lipopolysaccharides released from macrophages after the uptake of intact *E. coli in vitro*. *J. Immunol.*, **136**, 2924–9

31. Barclay, G. R., Scott, B. B., Wright, I. H., Rogers, P. N., Smith, D. G. E. and Poxton, I. R. (1989). Changes in anti-endotoxin-IgG antibody and endotoxaemia in three cases of Gram-negative septic shock. *Circ. Shock*, **29**, 93–106

32. Marks, J. D., Marks, C. B., Luce, J. M., Montgomery, A. B., Turner, J., Metz, C. A. and Murray, J. F. (1990). Plasma tumor necrosis factor in patients with septic shock. Mortality rate, incidence of adult respiratory distress syndrome, and effects of methylprednisolone administration. *Am. Rev. Respir. Dis.*, **141**, 94–7

33. Grob, P. J., Holch, M. and Brunner, W. (1987). Posttraumatisches/post-operatives Immundefektsyndrom. *Schweiz. Med. Wochenschr.*, **117**, 471–80

34. Goodwin, J. S. and Behrens, T. (1990). Humoral factors in immune sup-pression after injury. In Schlag, G., Redl, H. and Siegel, J. H. (eds.) *Shock, Sepsis, and Organ Failure*, pp. 329–49. (Berlin:Springer)

35. Cohen, J. and Glauser, M. P. (1991). Septic shock: treatment. *Lancet*, **338**, 736–9

36. Siegel, J. H. (1990). Multiple organ failure as a systemic disease of host-defense failure. In Schlag, G., Regl, H. and Siegel, J. H. (eds.) *Shock, Sepsis and Organ Failure*, pp. 627–38. (Berlin:Springer)

37. Heim, C. (1990). Operationsrisiko bei vorbestehenden allgemeinen Infekten und/oder Immunschwäche. *Ther. Umschau.*, **47**, 546–53

38. Chandra, R. K. (1989). Nutritional regulation of immunity and risk of infection in old age. *Immunology*, **67**, 141–7

39. Christou, N. V. (1989). Relationship between immune function and post-trauma morbidity and mortality. In Faist, E., Ninnemann, J. and Green, D. (eds.) *Immune Consequences of Trauma, Shock, and Sepsis. Mechanisms and Therapeutic Approaches*, pp. 357–62. (Berlin:Springer)

40. Barandun, S., Imbach, P., Kindt, H., Morell, A., Nydegger, U. E., Römer, J., Schneider, T., Sidiropoulos, D. and Skvaril, F. (eds.) (1981). *Der klinische Einsatz von Immunoglobulin (Gammaglobulin)*. (Basel:Sandoz)

41. Schwander, R., Hess, M. W., Keller, H. U. and Cottier, H. (1980). The post-natal development of lymph nodes in mice. *Immunobiol.*, **157**, 425–36

42. Luscieti, P., Hubschmid, T., Cottier, H., Hess, M. W. and Sobin, L. H. (1980). Human lymph node morphology as a function of age and site. *J. Clin. Pathol.*, **33**, 454–61
43. Duswald, K. H., Müller, K., Seifert, J. and Ring, J. (1980). Wirksamkeit von i.v. Gammaglobulin gegen bakterielle Infektionen chirurgischer Patienten. *Münch. Med. Wochenschr.*, **122**, 832–6
44. Baumgartner, J. D. (1991). Immunotherapy with antibodies to core lipopolysaccharide; a critical appraisal. *Infect. Dis. Clin. N. A.*, **5**, 915–27
45. Glinz, W., Grob, P. J., Nyedegger, U. E., Ricklin, T., Stamm, F., Stoffel, D. and Lasance, A. (1985). Polyvalent immunoglobulins for prophylaxis of bacterial infections in patients following multiple trauma. *Intens. Care Med.*, **11**, 288–94
46. Just, H. M., Metzger, M., Vogel, W. and Pelka, R. B. (1986). Einfluss einer adjuvanten Immunoglobulintherapie auf Infektionen bei Patienten einer operativen Intensiv-Therapie-Station. *Klin. Wochenschr.*, **64**, 245–56
47. DeSimone, C., Delogu, G. and Corbetta, G. (1988). Intravenous immuno-globulins in association with antibiotics: a therapeutic trial in septic intensive care unit patients. *Crit. Care Med.*, **16**, 23–6
48. Dominioni, L., Dionigi, R., Zanello, M., Chiaranda, M., Acquarolo, A., Ballabio, A. and Sguotti, C. (1991). Effects of high-dose IgG on survival of surgical patients with sepsis scores of 20 or greater. *Arch. Surg.*, **126**, 236–40
49. Garner, R. J. and Sacher, R. A. (eds.) (1988). *Intravenous Gammaglobulin Therapy*. (Arlington:Am. Assoc. Blood Banks)
50. McCabe, W. R., DeMaria, A. Jr, Berberich, H. and Johns, M. A. (1988). Immunization with rough mutants of *Salmonella minnesota*: protective activity of IgM and IgG antibody to the R595 (Re chemotype) mutant. *J. Infect. Dis.*, **158**, 291–300
51. Cafiero, F., Gipponi, M., Bonalumi, U., Piccardo, A., Sguotti, C. and Corbetta, G. (1992). Prophylaxis of infection with intravenous immuno-globulins plus antibiotic for patients at risk for sepsis undergoing surgery for colorectal cancer: results of a randomized, multicenter clinical trial. *Surgery*, **112**, 24–31
52. Nydegger, U. E. (1992). Immunoglobulins in antibacterial defense. In Cottier, H. and Kraft, R. (eds.) *Gut-Derived Infectious–Toxic Shock (GITS). Current Studies in Hematology and Blood Transfusion*, No. 59, pp. 146–62. (Basel:Karger)
53. Cottier, H., Ruchti, C. and Burkhardt, A. (1990). Adult respiratory distress syndrome due to an acute breach in the intestinal barrier. Should high-dose intravenous immunoglobulin therapy be tested? *Vox Sang.*, **58**, 311–23

54. Pilz, G., Class, I., Boekstegers, P., Pfeifer, A., Müller, U. and Werdan, K. (1991). *Pseudomonas* immunoglobulin therapy in patients with *Pseudomonas* sepsis and septic shock. In Homma, J. Y., Tanimoto, H., Holder, I. A., Hoiby, N. and Döring, G. (eds.) *Pseudomonas aeruginosa in Human Diseases, Antibiotic Chemotherapy*, Vol. 44, pp. 120–35. (Basel:Karger)

55. Cross, A. S., Sadoff, J. C. and Cryz, S. J. (1990). Vaccines against *Klebsiella* and *Pseudomonas* infections. In Woodrow, G. C. and Levine, M. M. (eds.) *New Generation Vaccines*, pp. 699–713. (New York:Marcel Dekker)

56. Tutschka, P. J. (1988). Gammaglobulin therapy in bone marrow transplantation. In Garner, R. J. and Sacher, R. A. (eds.) *Intravenous Gammaglobulin Therapy*, pp. 79–97. (Arlington:Am. Assoc. Blood Banks)

57. Baumgartner, J. D., Calandra, T. and Glauser, M. P. (1988). Intervention on Gram-negative bacterial disease by immunoglobulin therapy: reality or myth? In Krijnen, H. W., Strengers, P. F. W. and van Aken, W. G. (eds.) *Immunoglobulins*, pp. 191–205. (Amsterdam:Central Laboratory of the Netherlands Red Cross Blood Transfusion Service)

58. Baumgartner, J. D. (1990). Monoclonal anti-endotoxin antibodies for the treatment of Gram-negative bacteremia and septic shock. *Eur. J. Clin. Microbiol. Infect. Dis.*, **9**, 711–16

59. Tracey, K. J., Fong, Y., Hesse, D. G., Manogue, K. R., Lee, A. T., Kuo, G. C., Lowry, S. F. and Cerami, A. (1987). Anti-cachectin/TNF monoclonal antibodies prevent septic shock during lethal bacteraemia. *Nature (London)*, **330**, 662–4

60. Ziegler, E. J., Fisher, C. F., Sprung, C. L., Staube, R. C., Sadoff, J. C., Foulke, G. E., Wortel, C. H., Fink, M. P., Dellinger, R. P., Teng, N. N. H., Allen, I. E., Berger, H. J., Knatterud, G. L., LoBuglio, A. F., Smith, C. R. and HA-1A Sepsis Study Group (1991). Treatment of Gram-negative bacteremia and septic shock with HA-IA human monoclonal antibody against endotoxin. A randomized, double-blind, placebo-controlled trial. *N. Engl. J. Med.*, **324**, 429–36

61. Intravenous Immunoglobulin Collaborative Study Group (1992). Prophylactic intravenous administration of standard immune globulin as compared with core-lipopolysaccharide immune globulin in patients at high risk of postsurgical infection. *N. Engl. J. Med.*, **327**, 234–40

62. Baumgartner, J. D. (1991). Sepsis: la thérapie immunologique promet beaucoup (trop?). *Med. Hyg.*, **49**, 2702–9

63. Imbach, P., Hässig, A. and Cottier, H. (1992). Possibilities of immunoprophylaxis and immunotherapy in gut-derived infectious–toxic shock (GITS). In Cottier, H. and Kraft, R. (eds.) *Gut-Derived Infectious–Toxic Shock (GITS). Current Studies in Hematology and Blood Transfusion*, No. 59, pp. 301–23. (Basel:Karger)

3

Attenuation of complement immune damage by intravenous immunoglobulins

M. Basta, M. M. Frank and L. F. Fries

INTRODUCTION

Immunoglobulins modified for intravenous use were introduced into clinical practice a decade ago. Currently, these products are approved in the US for only two indications: first, primary immunodeficiency with hypogammaglobulinemia; and second, idiopathic thrombocytopenic purpura (ITP). However, it appears from numerous reports that intravenous immunoglobulin (IVIG) has a substantial short- and long-term therapeutic potential in a variety of immune disorders, but the underlying mechanisms of its beneficial effects are not understood.

Several theories have been introduced, such as competition of infused IVIG for macrophage Fc receptors, with the subsequent inhibition of IgG–Fc-mediated clearance[1,2]. Other theories include the modulation of autoantibody production by suppressive anti-idiotypic antibodies present in IVIG preparations[3] and direct effects on lymphoid cells, such as the decrease in helper : suppressor cell ratio in ITP[4] and Kawasaki disease[5] patients, and the arrest of maturation of peripheral blood B lymphocytes to plasma cells[6].

Our objective was to explore the possible interference of immunoglobulin molecules injected intravenously in high doses with the complement system. Our methodology encompassed two *in vivo* models of complement-dependent immune injury that are free of IgG–Fc interactions, and several *in vitro* complement uptake assays.

43

IN VIVO MODELS OF COMPLEMENT-DEPENDENT IMMUNE INJURY

Erythrocytes sensitized with IgM class antibodies are cleared from the circulation by the liver, both in humans and in guinea pigs[7]. The clearance curve has a characteristic shape: after initial hepatic sequestration at 5–15-min time points (which is presumably due to adhesion of the erythrocytes to Küpffer cells), a significant proportion of the detained cells are released back into the circulation, where they appear to survive normally.

We treated guinea pigs with a human IVIG preparation at 600 mg/kg for 2 consecutive days, and found that the clearance of IgM-sensitized guinea pig erythrocytes was significantly retarded compared to a control group of animals treated with saline (Figure 1). The effect was found to

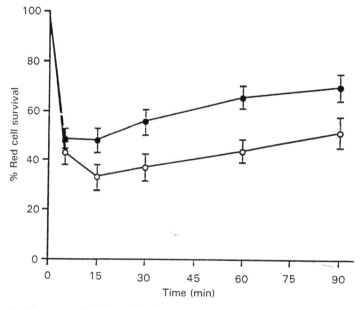

Figure 1 Clearance of IgM-sensitized guinea pig erythrocytes in guinea pigs treated with intravenous immunoglobulin (IVIG). The experimental group of animals (—●—, $n = 8$) was treated with the human IVIG at 600 mg/kg for 2 consecutive days. The parallel group of animals (—○—, $n = 8$) was treated with the same volume of saline. The survival of IgM-sensitized, ^{51}Cr-labelled guinea pig erythrocytes in the circulation of IVIG-treated animals was significantly prolonged relative to saline-treated animals. Data are means ± SEM. Reproduced with kind permission from reference 8

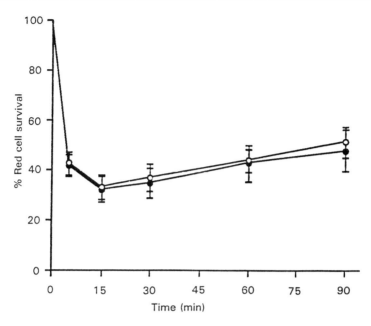

Figure 2 The effect of albumin on the clearance of IgM-sensitized erythrocytes. Four guinea pigs were treated with human albumin at 600 mg/kg for 2 consecutive days (—●—). Their average clearance curve was compared with that of the saline-infused animals (—○—) described in the legend to Figure 1. As shown, albumin failed to alter clearance of IgM target cells in comparison to saline. Data are means ± SEM. Reproduced with kind permission from reference 8

be specific for IVIG, since no change of target clearance was observed in parallel groups of animals treated with the same concentrations of human albumin (Figure 2)[8].

Forssman shock is a model of IgG-dependent complement-mediated acute tissue damage. It has been classified as a type II reaction using the system of Coombs and Gell[9]. These reactions are cytotoxic and caused by antibodies that recognize cellular antigens, with subsequent complement activation. Intravenous administration of anti-Forssman antiserum into a Forssman-positive animal such as a guinea pig, results in IgG antibody binding to Forssman antigen situated in the vascular endothelium of pulmonary capillaries, and the triggering of the complement cascade via the classical pathway. Subsequent necrosis and disintegration of the endothelial lining causes pulmonary edema, hemorrhage and death of the animal within minutes following the injection[10].

We found that IVIG treatment significantly prolonged survival and prevented death in 20% of guinea pigs subjected to otherwise lethal doses of anti-Forssman antiserum[11]. No control animal, treated with equivalent doses of albumin and/or maltose vehicle, survived Forssman shock. This effect, achieved with a treatment regimen similar to the one applied in human ITP (600 mg kg^{-1} day^{-1} for 3 days) was greatly enhanced by delivering the total dose as one slow injection of IVIG at 1800 mg/kg, 3 h before Forssman shock was elicited. Under these circumstances, the median duration of survival was increased five times and mortality was prevented in 38% (Figure 3). In the subsequent series of experiments, up to 75% of treated animals survived injections of lethal doses of anti-Forssman antiserum; a highly significant correlation of survival with human immunoglobulin dosage levels was found (not shown).

In both *in vivo* systems, therapy itself did not affect complement levels; C3 and CH$_{50}$ values remained unchanged after IVIG treatment relative

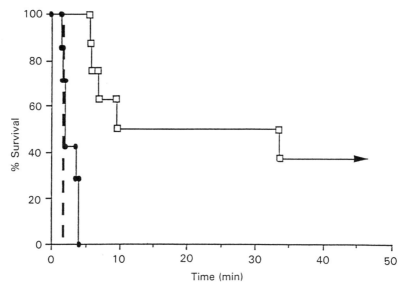

Figure 3 The effect of intravenous immunoglobulin (IVIG) treatment on survival in Forssman shock. Eight guinea pigs were injected with IVIG at 1800 mg/kg (—□—) while controls (—●—, *n* = 7) received 10% maltose supplemented with human albumin to yield 1800 mg/kg. Five animals (— — —) were completely untreated. 38% of guinea pigs treated with IVIG survived Forssman shock. All control animals (albumin-treated as well as untreated) died within 2 min following the provocation of Forssman shock. Reproduced with kind permission from reference 11

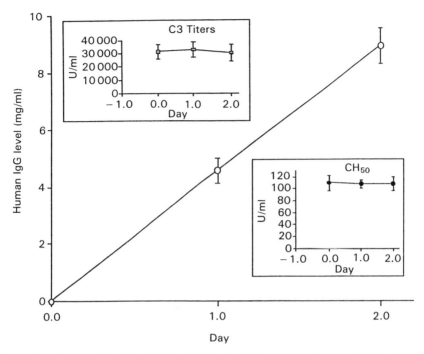

Figure 4 Human IgG levels and C3 and CH_{50} titers in intravenous immunoglobulin (IVIG)-treated guinea pigs. C3 titers, CH_{50} and the concentration of human IgG were determined in the sera of guinea pigs taken before (day 0), after 1 day (day 1) and after 2 days (day 2) of IVIG therapy at 600 mg/kg. Human IgG levels reached a value of 9 mg/ml on day 2. CH_{50} and C3 titers remained unchanged relative to pretreatment (day 0) values. Reproduced with kind permission from reference 8

to preinfusion (day 0) values, in spite of the steady increase of human IgG concentration in the sera of treated animals (Figure 4), indicating that the IVIG effect cannot be ascribed to a decrease in available plasma complement components. Similarly, the capacity to activate complement was not affected by the treatment: following provocation of Forssman shock, complement was consumed to the same extent in both IVIG-treated and control animals (not shown).

IN VITRO COMPLEMENT UPTAKE STUDIES

In order to more precisely elucidate the mechanism of the effect of IVIG on the complement system and to identify the steps along the classical complement cascade at which IVIG interferes, we developed several *in vitro* complement uptake assays, which consisted of the following:

(1) Washing and standardization of homologous erythrocytes;

(2) Sensitization of erythrocytes with IgG or IgM antierythrocyte antibodies (EA);

(3) Incubation of EA with serum supplemented with IVIG or appropriate control reagents (human albumin, buffer, maltose) at 37 °C;

(4) Taking aliquots of the mixture at certain times;

(5) Washing the aliquoted cells and incubating with appropriate radio-labelled anticomplement antibodies; and

(6) Quantitation of the uptake of complement fragments on to EA by determining counts/min using a gamma counter.

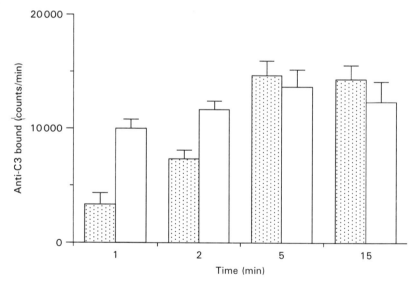

Figure 5 The effect of intravenous immunoglobulin (IVIG) on C3 uptake by IgM-sensitized guinea pig erythrocytes. IgM-sensitized guinea pig erythrocytes were incubated *in vitro* with undiluted serum from a guinea pig treated with human IVIG preparation (▣) and undiluted normal guinea pig serum (□). Aliquots were removed at various time points, and C3 uptake quantified using ^{125}I-labelled anti-guinea pig C3 antibody. Marked depression of C3 uptake was observed, compared with the uptake in normal serum control at early time points (1 and 2 min); at later time points such differences were no longer observed. Reproduced with kind permission from reference 8

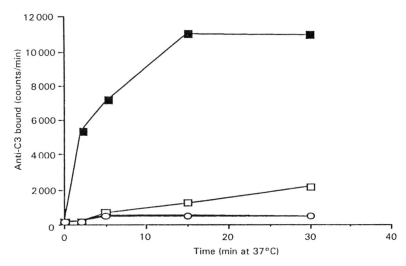

Figure 6 The effect of intravenous immunoglobulin (IVIG) on C3 uptake by IgG-sensitized guinea pig erythrocytes. IgG-sensitized guinea pig erythrocytes were incubated with normal guinea pig serum (—■—) and sera from animals treated with 600 mg/kg (—□—), 1200 mg/kg (—○—). C3 uptake was quantified by binding of ^{125}I-labelled anti-guinea pig C3 antibody, and was basically depressed to background values, even with the lowest IVIG dose. Reproduced with kind permission from reference 11

words, a marked inhibition of otherwise very rapid uptake of C3 by IgM-sensitized erythrocytes was observed at early time points (1 and 2 min). At 5 and 15 min the difference in respect to C3 uptake disappeared (Figure 5). On the other hand, almost complete inhibition of C3 uptake on to IgG-sensitized erythrocytes was obtained in an IVIG-treated animal's serum (Figure 6).

Because there are many similarities between C3 and C4 molecules, especially in terms of activation through an internal thiol–ester bond, we next examined the influence of IVIG on C4 uptake on to sensitized erythrocytes[12]. IVIG inhibited C4 uptake on to IgM-sensitized guinea pig erythrocytes by approximately 20%. The effect was much more pronounced when IgG-sensitized targets were used; inhibition of 50% was observed at all time points (Figure 7). Reduced C4 uptake on to sensitized homologous erythrocytes was also found in the serum from a patient treated with IVIG; in comparison with serum from the same patient before IVIG therapy, C4 uptake was decreased to almost background level (Figure 8).

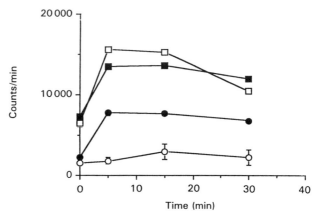

Figure 7 The effect of intravenous immunoglobulin (IVIG) on C4 uptake by IgG-sensitized guinea pig erythrocytes. Guinea pig erythrocytes were sensitized with anti-guinea pig antibodies of IgG class and then incubated with normal guinea pig serum (NGPS) diluted 1 : 4 (—■—), NGPS substituted with 10 mg/tube of human IVIG (—●—), NGPS with 10 mg/tube of human albumin for i.v. use (—□—), C4 uptake by non-sensitized guinea pig erythrocytes (so-called 'E' control) (—○—). Aliquots were removed at different time points for C4 uptake quantification by radiolabelled anti-guinea pig C4 IgG antibody. C4 uptake inhibition of 50% was observed at all time points. Reproduced with kind permission from reference 12

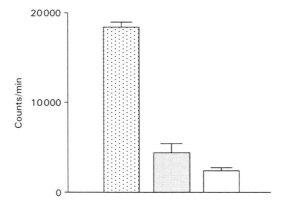

Figure 8 The effect of serum from an intravenous immunoglobulin (IVIG)-treated patient on C4 binding to sensitized human erythrocytes. Serum samples were collected from a patient before and after 3-day therapy with IVIG at 600 mg/kg. Human erythrocytes were sensitized with rabbit anti-human red cell IgG antibody and incubated with the undiluted serum from a patient before (⊞) and after (□) IVIG therapy; non-sensitized erythrocytes (□) were incubated with autologous human serum. After a 5-min incubation at 37 °C, aliquots of cells were removed for C4 uptake quantification by anti-human C4 antibody labelled with ^{125}I. In the presence of post-IVIG serum, C4 uptake was almost completely blocked. Reproduced with kind permission from reference 12

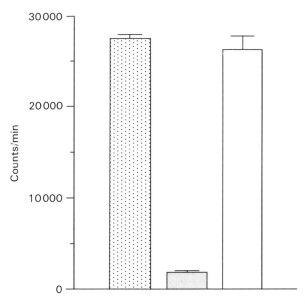

Figure 9 C1q uptake in the presence of serum from a patient before and after intravenous immunoglobulin (IVIG) therapy. Sensitized human erythrocytes were incubated with the serum before (□) and after (▣) IVIG therapy; non-sensitized erythrocytes (▨) were incubated with autologous human serum. After a 5-min incubation at 30 °C, aliquots of cells were removed and C1q uptake was quantified by ^{125}I-labelled anti-C1q antibody. C1q uptake was not depressed in the presence of post-IVIG serum. Reproduced with kind permission from reference 13

One possible and logical explanation for the observed phenomenon of C3/C4 uptake inhibition could be the blockade of the first step of the classical complement activation pathway or recognition phase, which consists of C1q binding to sensitized erythrocytes. To examine that possibility, we investigated the ability of human serum containing high doses of IVIG to deposit the recognition subunit of the first complement component on to targets[13]. Such serum did not demonstrate reduced C1q binding to targets as determined by radiolabelled antihuman C1q antibody uptake (Figure 9). At increasing doses of sensitizing antibody C1q uptake decreased proportionally; however, at all antibody dilution points C1q uptake was not significantly different in the serum with IVIG as compared with normal serum (Figure 10). Based on the above data, we concluded that IVIG did not interfere with the recognition step of the classical complement pathway.

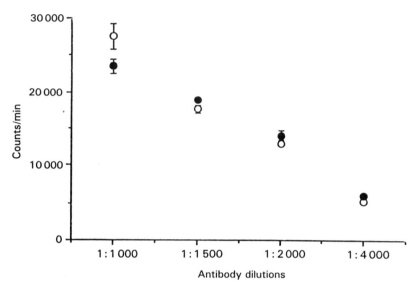

Figure 10 C1q uptake on to human red blood cells sensitized with different dilutions of antihuman erythrocyte antibody. Human erythrocytes were sensitized with antihuman erythrocyte IgG antibody diluted 1:1000, 1:1500, 1:2000 and 1:4000, and subsequently incubated with autologous human serum with and without 5 mg/tube of intravenous immunoglobulin (IVIG). After a 15-min incubation, aliquots of cells were removed and C1q uptake was quantitated by the uptake of radiolabelled antihuman C1q IgG antibody. At all dosage points, serum with added IVIG (O) manifested C1q uptake equal to the serum without IVIG (●). Reproduced with kind permission from reference 13

PATIENT STUDIES

Several patient studies were performed in order to substantiate the conclusions drawn from the studies in the guinea pig system. Blood cells from patients with complement-dependent immune disorders before and following IVIG therapy were subjected to a series of *in vitro* experiments. We were interested in the number of C3 molecules on the surface of these autoantibody-sensitized cells, since our hypothesis was that high serum levels of IVIG could protect cells newly produced in the bone marrow and entering the circulation from the deposition of activated C3 molecules; if this really happens *in vivo*, then one would expect a decrease of C3 molecules on the surface of blood cells in post-IVIG samples relative to pretreatment values.

We first studied patients with autoimmune hemolytic anemia (AIHA). In two adult patients we found a significant decrease of C3 molecules on their red cells after IVIG therapy, as determined by the uptake of radio-labelled polyclonal antihuman C3 antibody. Similarly, percent–specific incorporation of radiolabelled monoclonal anti–C3d, and anti–C3c on to erythrocytes of children treated with standard doses of IVIG was significantly reduced, compared with pretreatment incorporation (not shown). Consistent with these findings in AIHA patients were the results of the study that involved a patient with autoimmune neutrope-nia and thrombocytopenia; after one dose of IVIG at 400 mg/kg, the number of C3 molecules (detected by ^{125}I labelled anti–C3 antibody) decreased by 15% and the number of platelets increased by 70% relative to preinfusion values.

Red cells from two patients suffering from paroxysmal nocturnal hemoglobinuria (PNH) were protected from *in vitro* (acid) lysis by the addition of 20 mg/ml of IVIG to the test tube, compared to the test tube without added IVIG (Table 1).

Table 1   Inhibition of acid lysis of erythrocytes from paroxysmal nocturnal hemoglobinuria (PNH) patients by addition of intravenous immunoglobulin (IVIG)

	Lysis (%)	
Patient	*–IVIG*	*+IVIG*
KM	49	10
JC	87	54

CONCLUSION

Our data suggest that supraphysiological levels of IVIG act by preventing C3/C4 fragments from binding to target cells, i.e. high-dose IVIG might provide a 'sink' that could divert these highly proinflammatory com-plement fragments away from sites of immunological tissue damage. Complement is known to play a major role in the pathogenesis of many debilitating and life-threatening diseases in humans. Therapy for these disorders is inefficient and consists mainly of prolonged glucocorticoid administration, which often causes serious side-effects. Our results suggest that infusion of one very large dose of IVIG may be a reasonable approach to modulate acute complement-dependent tissue damage in humans. In addition to diseases such as acute glomerulonephritis, vasculitis syndrome, hemolytic episodes in AIHA and PNH, IVIG could prove to be effective in a variety of states mediated by cleavage products formed during complement activation (acute allergic reactions, heart muscle damage following the initial insult during infarction, rapid multiplication of tumor cells in terminal stages of some malignancies). We hope that a large number of patients suffering from complement-mediated diseases will benefit from this new, much safer and effective therapeutic approach.

REFERENCES

1. Kurlander, R. J., Ellison, D. M. and Hall, J. (1984). The blockade of Fc receptor-mediated clearance of immune complexes *in vivo* by monoclonal antibody (2.4G2) directed against Fc receptors on murine leukocytes. *J. Immunol.*, **133**, 855

2. Fehr, J., Hoffman, V. and Kappeler, U. (1982). Transient reversal of thrombocytopenia in idiopathic thrombocytopenic purpura by high-dose intravenous γ-globulin. *N. Engl. J. Med.*, **306**, 1254

3. Rossi, F., Sultan, Y. and Kazatchkine, M. D. (1986). Spontaneous and therapeutic suppression of autoimmune response to factor VIII by anti-idiotypic antibodies. In Morell, A. and Nydegger, U. E. (eds.) *Clinical Use of Intravenous Immunoglobulins*, p. 421. (London:Academic Press)

4. Dammacco, F., Iodice, G. and Campobasso, N. (1986). Treatment of adult patients with idiopathic thrombocytopenic purpura with intravenous immunoglobulin: effects on circulating T-cell subsets and PWM-induced antibody synthesis *in vitro*. *Br. J. Haematol.*, **62**, 125

5. Leung, D. Y., Burns, J. C., Newberg, J. W. and Geha, R. S. (1987). Reversal of lymphocyte activation *in vivo* in the Kawasaki syndrome by intravenous gammaglobulin. *J. Clin. Invest.*, **79**, 468

6. Durandy, A., Fisher, A. and Griscelli, C. (1981). Dysfunctions of pokeweed mitogen-stimulated T and B lymphocyte responses induced by gammaglobulin therapy. *J. Clin. Invest.*, **67**, 867

7. Frank, M. M. (1977). Pathophysiology of immune hemolytic anemia. *Ann. Intern. Med.*, **87**, 210

8. Basta, M., Langlois, P. F., Marques, M., Frank, M. M. and Fries, L. F. (1989). High-dose intravenous immunoglobulin modifies complement-mediated *in vivo* clearance. *Blood*, **74**, 326

9. Coombs, R. R. A., and Gell, P. G. H. (1975). Classification of allergic reactions responsible for clinical hypersensitivity and disease. In Gell, P. G. H., Coombs, R. R. A. and Lachman, P. J. (eds.) *Clinical Aspects of Immunology*, (London:Blackwell Scientific)

10. Taichman, N. S., Creighton, M., Stephenson, A. and Tsai, C. C. (1972). Ultrastructure of pulmonary vascular lesions produced by Forssman anti-serum in guinea pigs. *Immunology*, **22**, 93

11. Basta, M., Kirshbom, P., Frank, M. M. and Fries, L. F. (1989). Mechanism of therapeutic effect of high-dose intravenous immunoglobulin. Attenuation of acute, complement-dependent immune damage in a guinea pig model. *J. Clin. Invest.*, **84**, 1974–81

12. Basta, M., Frics, L. F. and Frank, M. M. (1991). High-dose intravenous Ig inhibits *in vitro* uptake of C4 fragments onto sensitized erythrocytes. *Blood*, **77**, 376–80

13. Basta, M., Fries, L. F. and Frank, M. M. (1991). High doses of intravenous immunoglobulin do not affect the recognition phase of the classical complement pathway. *Blood*, **78**, 700–2

4

Control of spontaneous hemorrhage without normalization of hemostatic defect: an endothelial effect?

E. Rewald

The following clinical observations led us to hypothesize that the permeability of endothelia for the passage of red cells may be influenced in some way by IgG. Since it was shown that most cases of autoimmune thrombocytopenic purpura (ATP) respond satisfactorily to high-dose intravenous immunoglobulin therapy (IVIG), the other immune cytopenias have been treated in the same way. Whereas the results in neutropenia are usually acceptable, those in hemolytic anemia have been controversial. Rhesus hemolytic disease of the newborn is provoked by a similar mechanism, except that on the one hand the red cells which sensitize the mother have to cross the placental barrier, and on the other hand the maternal antibodies must invade the fetal bloodstream. As it is known, during subsequent incompatible pregnancies, the antibody synthesis rebounds, increasing the danger of stillbirth. Treating the mother with high doses of intravenous IgG seems to improve fetal outcome, provided that the maternal antibody titer is not excessively high. Our findings began in 1964[1,2], and have since been confirmed by other authors[3-5]. When IVIG administration is started at the beginning of the second trimester of pregnancy, the antibody titer does not rise further and even tends to decrease[1,4,5]. This suggests that one of the IVIG mechanisms seems to be the prevention of maternal antibody booster reaction (Figures 1–3). Paradoxically, Petri and colleagues[6] reported on the work of Kerényi, regarding a procedure in which anti-D IgG was given to pregnant

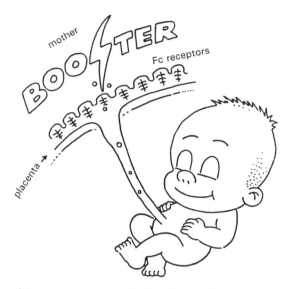

Figure 1 Effect of the placental passage of fetal red blood cells on the maternal antibody titer

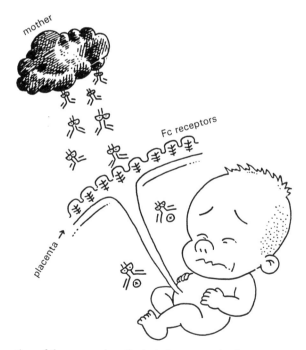

Figure 2 Prevention of the maternal antibody influence on the fetus

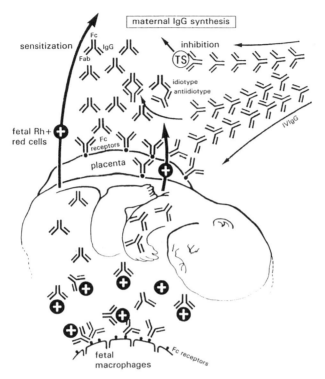

Figure 3 Other possible mechanisms of an effect of intravenous immunoglobulin (IVIG) therapy in Rh(D)-incompatibility. TS, T suppressor cell

women who were already Rh(D) sensitized. IgG blocked the progress of the immunization in 88% of 67 cases, and the prospects for the endangered fetus were much improved.

Like Salama and colleagues[7], we have observed that high-dose IVIG, and also much smaller doses of anti-Rh(D) preparations, with high concentration of aggregates of IgG, may prevent spontaneous thrombocytopenic hemorrhage (Figure 4) even in the absence of an increase in the number of platelets. So, during the last 6 years, we have successfully managed not only patients with ATP whose platelets failed to respond to IVIG therapy, but also those who became thrombocytopenic due to aplastic anemia, myelodysplasia and heavy chemotherapy, with platelets well below the critical level of 10 000/μl. Initially, we suspected that the prolonged period free of hemorrhagic complications was caused by a qualitative improvement in the platelets, although due to their

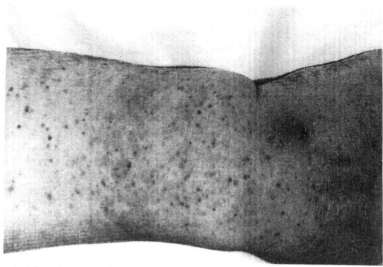

Figure 4 Thrombocytopenic purpura

low concentration we were unable to perform functional tests. As hematopoietic cells remain defective, a functional recovery of the scarce platelets causing the remission of bleeding tendency seems to be unlikely. Of course, isolated cases cannot test the efficacy of a treatment. Spontaneous hemorrhage is variable, and might be subject to a placebo effect, but this should have been more remarkable during the initial period of therapy, whereas, according to our observations, there was a delay in the disappearance of bleeding manifestations. Among the abundant literature on hemorrhage, the scarcity of references concerning the mechanism of apparently spontaneous petechiae and bruises is noteworthy. The subject seems to us very important, because there are a number of patients with chronic risky bleeding tendency who become refractory to platelet transfusions, and who have to be maintained over years somehow protected from fatal hemorrhagic complications[8,9]. It has been suggested that an increased vascular resistance and hemostasis may explain why bleeding sometimes diminishes within a day or two after starting corticosteroid therapy for ATP, well before platelet counts begin to rise[10]. Also, as noted by Proctor[11], during the administration of α-interferon in ATP, the bleeding tendency was reduced even though platelet counts did not rise.

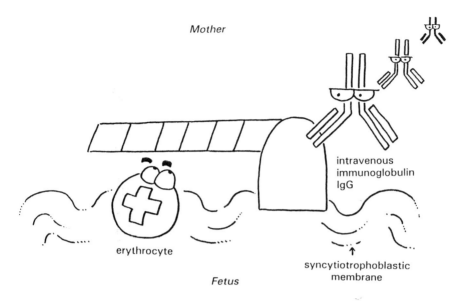

Figure 5 Possible preventive effect of intravenous immunoglobulin on the passage of fetal red cells

Briefly, in the search for an explanation to our observations, I would like to suggest the possibility that a direct or indirect effect of IgG preparations on the red cell 'porosity' of the vascular compartment be explored. This notion is in line with a possible reduction or even abolition of the usual transplacental passage of fetal erythrocytes (Figure 5), thus failing to boost maternal antibody synthesis. IgG therapy may improve not only the placental barrier, but also prevent red cell leakage through the capillary endothelial wall of the peripheral circulation that causes petechiae and bruises. In cases of acquired hemophilia due to an autoantibody to factor VIII, which responded to high doses of IVIG, the apparently spontaneous hemorrhages disappeared even before the factor VIII: C concentration had increased[12,13]. The putative effect on permeability may also reduce the passage of anti-Rh(D) antibodies to the fetus. All this is very hard to prove until double-blind placebo-controlled studies document these clinical impressions conclusively. The clinical endpoint must be validated for IVIG and anti-Rh(D) immunoglobulin.

REFERENCES

1. Rewald, E. and Suringar, F. (1965). Substitutive–inhibitory γ-globulin therapy as prevention of stillbirth in Rh incompatibility. *Acta. Haematol.*, **34**, 209–14

2. Rewald, E. and Suringar, F. (1968). Tolerance of intravenous γ-globulin. *Bibl. Haematol.*, **29**, 337–9

3. Berlin, G., Selbing, A. and Ryden, G. (1985). Rhesus haemolytic disease treated with high-dose intravenous immunoglobulin. *Lancet*, **1**, 1153

4. De la Cámara, C., Arrieta, R., González, A., Iglesias, E. and Omeñaca, F. (1988). High-dose intravenous immunoglobulin as the sole prenatal treatment of severe Rh immunization. *N. Engl. J. Med.*, **318**, 519–20

5. Margulies, M., Voto, L. S., Mathet, E. and Margulies M. (1991). High-dose intravenous IgG for the treatment of severe rhesus alloimmunization. *Vox Sang.*, **61**, 181–8

6. Petri, I. B., Lórincz, A. and Berek, I. (1984). Detection of Fc-receptor-blocking antibodies in anti-Rh(D) hyperimmune gammaglobulin. *Lancet*, **2**, 1478–9

7. Salama, A., Kiefel, V., Amberg, R. and Mueller-Eckhardt, C. (1984). Treatment of autoimmune thrombocytopenic purpura with Rhesus antibodies (anti-Rho (D)). *Blut*, **49**, 29–34

8. Rewald, E. (1987). Repeated low doses of anti-Rhesus gammaglobulin in aplastic anaemia. *Lancet*, **2**, 795

9. Rewald, E. (1990). A vascular effect of IgG therapy may prevent transplacental red cell leakage and spontaneous thrombocytopenic haemorrhages. *Med. Hypoth.*, **33**, 193–5

10. Linker, C. (1988). Blood. In Schroeder, S. A., Krupp, M. A. and Tierney, L. M. (eds.) *Current Medical Diagnosis and Treatment 1988*, pp. 325–7, (Norwalk, Ct:Appleton & Lange)

11. Proctor, S. J. (1990). *Alpha Interferons in the Management of Idiopathic Thrombocytopenia.* Shering-Plough Alpha Interferon Monograph XIV

12. Rewald, E. Intravenous immunoglobulin and spontaneous hemorrhage in a case of Factor VIII inhibitor. (Abstract 1596, presented at the 24th Congress of the International Society of Haematology, London, 1992.) *Br. J. Haematol.*, (Special Issue)

13. Annetta, I., Otaso, J., Nucifora, E., Apezteguía, C. and Gioseffi, O. (1992). Inhibidor de factor VIII post-parto: presentación de 2 casos. *4a Reunión Científica (1992). Soc. Arg. Hematology*

5

Clinical results of high-dose immunoglobulin administration in severely septic surgical patients

L. Dominioni, R. Dionigi, R. Gennari and M. Besozzi

Infectious complications continue to be a major cause of morbidity and mortality in surgical patients in spite of improved intensive care techniques and multimodal therapy. The fatal outcome of sepsis usually results from progressive multiple organ failure or from septic shock.

Several studies have indicated that immunological alterations occur in severely septic patients, which may in part be the reason for their inability to control infection. Critical surgical and polytraumatized patients present numerous cellular and humoral disturbances, leading to decreased organic defenses against infection. Impaired phagocytosis and defective opsonic function in the serum of severely septic patients have been documented[1,2]. It has been shown that serum IgG levels are either within the normal range or supranormal in septic patients; however, IgG levels were documented to decrease in non-survivors and to increase in survivors. IgG with intact Fc were shown to enhance opsonization and phagocytosis *in vitro*[3]. In order to determine the mechanisms of bacterial opsonization by immunoglobulins, recent studies, carried out using antibody-deficient human serum, have examined complement consumption and polymorphonuclear leukocyte (PMNL) membrane receptor-mediated internalization of a variety of bacteria opsonized by immunoglobulin. These studies showed that immunoglobulin alone did not consume complement, and had no opsonic activity for the organisms tested; however, when bacteria were preopsonized in immunoglobulin, significant amounts of complement were consumed and the uptake and killing of bacteria occurred. These data indicate that immunoglobulin alone does not contribute to effective bacterial opsonization, whereas optimal opsonic activity of immuno-globulin is mediated through complement activation. Animal studies have shown that the prophylactic administration of intact immuno-globulin decreases mortality from burn wound sepsis.

Other recent studies have shown that human antiserum to the lipopoly-saccharide core can reduce mortality from gram-negative septicemia in severe sepsis; in order to develop a more specific therapy of endotoxemia, human monoclonal IgM antibody that binds selectively to the lipid A domain of endotoxin (HA-1A) has been proposed; it has been shown that HA-1A is safe and can be used for the treatment of septic patients with gram-negative bacteremia, including those with septic shock[4].

In the surgical intensive care unit (ICU) severe infections are fre-quently observed arising from bacterial contamination at the moment of trauma or operation, or from invasive procedures. Major trauma and major surgery cause a decrease in bactericidal activity, a contributing factor in the increased sepsis rate. Clinical studies have been carried out to verify whether early intravenous immunoglobulin (IVIG) adminis-tration can effectively prevent surgical and post-traumatic sepsis, and data obtained suggest that early high-dose IVIG administration in ICU patients reduces the number of positive cultures, and also the incidence of sepsis and death[5,6].

In spite of these favorable experimental and clinical results, the effect of IVIG therapy in septic patients has never been unequivocally assessed, because it has proved difficult to perform studies with com-parable groups of septic individuals. In recent years, scoring systems for measuring the severity of surgical infections have been developed[7,8]; these methods can be used in controlled clinical trials to provide groups of patients with comparable severity of sepsis.

In order to assess whether high-dose IVIG can reduce sepsis-related mortality in severely septic, high-risk surgical patients undergoing intensive care treatment, we carried out a prospective, randomized, double-blind, placebo-controlled multicenter study in the surgical ICUs at the Universities of Varese, Bologna, Pavia and Brescia[9]. A total of 62 patients of both sexes admitted to the ICU for treatment of severe surgical infections were prospectively entered into this study on the day

(day 0 of the study) when their sepsis score reached 20 or greater. This level of sepsis score was selected to identify patients with a very high mortality risk[10]. We excluded patients from the study if they had had recent immunosuppressive treatment, a history of high-dose IVIG administration during the previous month, or other characteristics that would confound the interpretation of results.

The patient population studied included a wide variety of underlying diseases (perforation of hollow viscus, multiple trauma, splanchnic vascular disease, pancreatitis, extrasplanchnic vascular disease, intestinal obstruction) and septic complications (peritonitis, wound infection, pneumonia, septicemia, abscess, urinary tract infection.

Conventional multimodal therapy for the septic conditions was promptly instituted in all these patients. The clinical course of all patients was followed, recording their sepsis score at 3–5-day intervals until either they were discharged from the ICU or died. The causes of death were recorded and classified as due to multiple organ failure (three or more organs/systems failures), to septic shock (tissue hypoperfusion and refractory circulatory failure) or as not related to sepsis. In addition, patients randomly received intravenous administration of either polyvalent IgG with stabilized Fc subunits (Sandoglobulin®, Sandoz) (IVIG-treated patients) at the doses indicated in Table 1, or human albumin in 5% dextrose in water as placebo (controls).

Table 1 Dosage of IVIG for treatment of severe surgical infection

Patient weight	Dosage (g)		
	Day 0	*Day 1*	*Day 5*
≥ 50 kg	24	24	12
< 50 kg	18	18	12

After 62 patients had entered the protocol, the study was ended; it was found that 29 patients had received IVIG and 33 patients had received placebo. Group comparison between IVIG-treated patients and controls showed no significant differences in underlying disease or types of

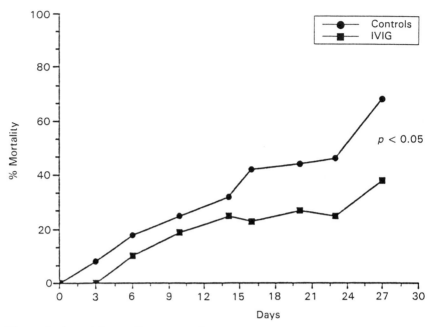

Figure 1 Actuarial mortality curves of intravenous immunoglobulin (IVIG)-treated and control patients

septic complications, and the number of infectious foci per patient. The mean sepsis scores at the beginning of ICU treatment were similar in both IVIG-treated and control patients (24 ± 4 and 24 ± 3; non-significant).

Analysis of the results indicated a significantly lower mortality ($p < 0.05$) in the IVIG-treated group: 11 of 29 patients died (38%), whereas in the control group 22 of 33 patients died (67%). The actuarial mortality curves in IVIG-treated patients and in control patients are illustrated in Figure 1. The causes of death in all patients were either septic shock or multiple organ failure, except in one patient. IVIG-treated patients presented a significantly lower death rate from septic shock, compared to controls (7% versus 33%; $p < 0.05$). Among all causes of death in IVIG-treated patients, septic shock accounted for 18% (2 of 11 patients). In control patients septic shock accounted for 50% (11 of 22) of all causes of death. The percentage of IVIG-treated and control patients who died of multiple organ failure was similar

(31% and 30%, respectively). Thus, the reduced mortality of patients treated with high-dose IVIG in our study was due to a significantly lower incidence of lethal septic shock.

In another study, IVIG was given prophylactically to surgical patients at risk of infection, and was also shown to reduce the incidence of postoperative infections[5]. Moreover, the incidence of pneumonia in multiple trauma patients was significantly reduced by the prophylactic use of large doses of IVIG[6].

Although it was suggested that high-dose IVIG administration can be deleterious to the reticuloendothelial system (RES), resulting in RES blockade with exacerbation of infecting processes, the results of our study do not suggest that this occurs. The mechanism by which the administration of high-dose IVIG improves the survival of severely septic surgical patients can be only tentatively hypothesized; it may be speculated that the opsonophagocytosis defects reported in septic patients are restored by high-dose IVIG.

We carried out another study in a series of septic patients with a broad range of severity of infections, to elucidate to what extent defects of opsonophagocytosis actually occur in septic patients, and to assess whether alterations of bacterial phagocytosis could be reversed by different doses of polyvalent IgG (Sandoglobulin®, Sandoz). The results of this study indicate that the polymorphonuclear leukocytes (PMNL) of septic patients present a significant depression in bacterial phagocytosis ($p < 0.001$) compared to healthy controls. However, phagocytosis is not altered to the same extent in all septic patients; in fact, we observed a significant correlation ($p < 0.001$) between sepsis score and deficiency of phagocytosis, indicating that only the very severely septic patients present a critically low bacterial phagocytosis[11]. The same study indicated that the defect of phagocytosis can be partly reversed by polyvalent IgG, with a dose-dependent effect. In patients with severe sepsis (sepsis score > 17), in whom PMNL phagocytosis was markedly depressed as compared to controls, only the administration of a high dose of IgG (≥ 0.4 g/kg) could reverse phagocytosis to near-normal levels.

In conclusion, the results of our studies indicate that, in severely septic patients, the deficit of PMNL phagocytosis can be partly reversed by high-dose polyvalent IgG; this may be a mechanism to explain the potential benefit of such therapy in the treatment of septic shock and life-threatening infections.

REFERENCES

1. Nishijima, M. K. *et al.* (1986). Serial changes in cellular immunity of septic patients with multiple organ system failure. *Crit. Care Med.*, **14**, 87–91
2. Alexander, J. W. *et al.* (1979). A comparison of immunologic profiles and their influence on bacteremia in surgical patients with a high risk of infection. *Surgery*, **86**, 94–104
3. Fisher, G. I. (1983). Functional antibacterial activity of human intravenous immunoglobulin preparation: *in vitro* and *in vivo* studies. *Vox Sang.*, **44**, 296–9
4. Ziegler, E. *et al.* (1991). Treatment of Gram-negative bacteremia and septic shock with HA-1A human monoclonal antibody against endotoxin. *N. Engl. J. Med.*, **324**, 429–36
5. Mao, P. *et al.* (1989). Early administration of intravenous immunoglobulins in the prevention of surgical and posttraumatic sepsis: a double-blind, randomized, clinical trial. *Surg. Res. Commun.*, **5**, 93–8
6. Glinz, W. *et al.* (1985). Polyvalent immunoglobulins for prophylaxis of bacterial infections in patients following multiple trauma. *Intens. Care Med.*, **11**, 288–94
7. Elebute, E. A. and Stoner, H. B. (1983). The grading of sepsis. *Br. J. Surg.*, **70**, 29–31
8. Dominioni, L. *et al.* (1987). The grading of sepsis and the assessment of its prognosis in the surgical patients: a review. *Surg. Res. Commun.*, **1**, 1–11
9. Dominioni, L. *et al.* (1991). Effects of high-dose IgG on survival of surgical patients with sepsis score of 20 or greater. *Arch. Surg.*, **126**, 236–40
10. Dominioni, L. *et al.* (1987). Sepsis score and acute phase protein response as predictors of outcome in septic surgical patients. *Arch. Surg.*, **122**, 141–6
11. Dominioni, L. *et al.* (1992). High-dose IG in severely septic surgical patients: effects on phagocytosis. *J. Roy. Coll. Surg. Edin.*, **37**, 275–6

6

Neonatal sepsis

F. Ramírez Osío

In the neonatal period there is a greater risk of infection than at any other time in life. Sepsis is one of the main causes of morbidity and mortality, with an incidence of 1–5 cases every 1000 live births registered, the mortality rate being constantly high (20–75%)[1,2]. This variability range is inversely related to gestational age, associated with immune deficits (impairment of natural barriers, decreased complement levels, low antibody titers, impaired lymphoid cell populations, impaired granulocyte production and functioning) plus a longer time of exposure to infectious agents in the nursery[3,4]. In spite of great advances in neonatal care, and the development of new antibiotics, newborn infants continue to die after failure of their natural and acquired defense mechanisms. The newborn child, who has lived in a sterile environment *in utero*, suddenly meets a series of bacteria in the mother's vagina (*Group B streptococcus, Escherichia coli, Listeria monocytogenes, Hemophilus influenzae* spp.) and can be infected before or during delivery (maternal infection, amnio-chorionic inflammation, premature rupture of membrane (PRM), meconium aspiration). Infection can present early, before the fifth day of life; this can be more serious and have an earlier onset in preterm infants, as well as being a late infection that appears in full-term and heavier premature babies; there is also vertical transmission due to the above-mentioned bacteria or a community infection due to organisms such as *Staphylococcus aureus* or *Group A streptococcus*. Babies also run the risk of infection from hospital personnel. In very low birth weight premature infants who must stay in hospital for more than a month, the mode of transmission can be vertical (*E. coli, Candida* spp., *Group B steptococcus* and enterococcus) or hospital-acquired (coagulase–negative staphylococcus, resistant species of *Staphylococcus aureus, Pseudomonas* spp., *Serratia* spp., etc.). In this group, clinical manifestations are variable and generally subtle, with a weak inflammatory response[5].

When different factors of the immune system are deficient, infection spreads, causing systemic damage and death. Among the different factors involved we must mention natural barriers, frequently overcome by resuscitating procedures, placing of catheters or sampling. In the neonatal period the skin is anatomically and functionally immature; permeability is increased, there is a diminution of melanin production, vesicle formation increases, pH is higher and there is a lower production of cholesterol and fatty acids. There are other modes of entry related to the umbilical area and birth trauma. In the gastrointestinal tract, diminished peristalsis in preterm infants, higher gastric pH, lower secretion of bile acids and IgA are all predisposing factors that increase the risk of infection. Other factors are a respiratory mucous membrane with less ciliary epithelium, and diminished saliva secretion[3].

Once the germ comes into contact with the organism, the immune and cellular responses occur with the recognition of self or foreign antigens: the immune response signals through cytokines released (tumor necrosis factor (TNF), interleukin-6 (IL-6)) by the macrophages involved (monocytes, macrophages of the marginal area, spleen, lymphatic nodes, Küpffer cells, microglial cells and Langerhans cells) and other cells without phagocytic activity, such as dendritic cells, astrocytes, T and B lymphocytes etc., and by the acute-phase activation response (C-reactive protein, fibrinogen, transferrin, etc.). The presence of specific antibodies against the organism fascilitates this response, favoring opsonization via Fc or through complement fragment C3b. If antibody is absent, the onset of its production must wait for antigen processing, which is recognized to be associated with major histocompatibility complex class I and II and the chain of events of the immune response, where T lymphocytes plus IL-2 and IL-4 participate, for these immune cells and mediators allow the formation of a clone of B and plasma cells, producing IgM as a primary response and IgG as a secondary response, specific for the antigen determining its production. These antibodies favor opsonophagocytosis, either directly or through complement activation. Simultaneously there is a stimulus for a medullary response to produce and release functioning leukocytes (chemotaxis C5a–C3a–granulocyte–macrophage colony-stimulating factor (GM-CSF)), which tend to eliminate the infectious agent with no damage to the child, thanks to their own immune mechanisms or the intervention of the physician[6,7]. The pathogenesis of sepsis is illustrated in Figure 1.

Innate or acquired impairment of the neonate's immune system has been thoroughly demonstrated in animal experiments and in humans; it has also been shown that its replacement improves the survival of the affected infant[8]. Thus, we found that complement (opsonins, chemoattractive anaphylatoxins) is diminished and opsonization is impaired, making more difficult the elimination of pathogens such as type 3 *Group B streptococcus*, which requires the specific capsular antibody for activation, and *E. coli* with K1 in its membrane, which requires the specific antibody for the activation of the classical route, avoiding meningeal invasion and neutrophil depletion in the bone marrow[9]. Diminished fibronectin impairs the adherence of opsonized germs to monocytes or macrophages[10].

With regard to phagocytes, many researchers have demonstrated significant *in vitro* alterations of neutrophil function in the neonate which are more serious in those suffering from stress or sepsis[11], specifically diminution of:

(1) Capacity of deformability,

(2) Chemotaxis,

(3) Phagocytosis,

(4) C3bi receptor expression,

(5) Polymorphonuclear leukocyte (PMN) adherence, and

(6) Bactericidal ability and alterations in oxidative metabolism.

As to the size of the proliferation pool, there is a diminution in granulo-cyte–macrophage colony-forming units (25% of cells), with almost maximum proliferating ability (75%)[12,13]. GM-CSF is produced in lesser amounts[14], involving the production, release and function of neutrophils. The accelerated exit of neutrophils from the pool, being rapidly utilized during infection, makes the neonate prone to significant neutropenia ($<1800/mm^3$). The neutrophil pool is diminished by about

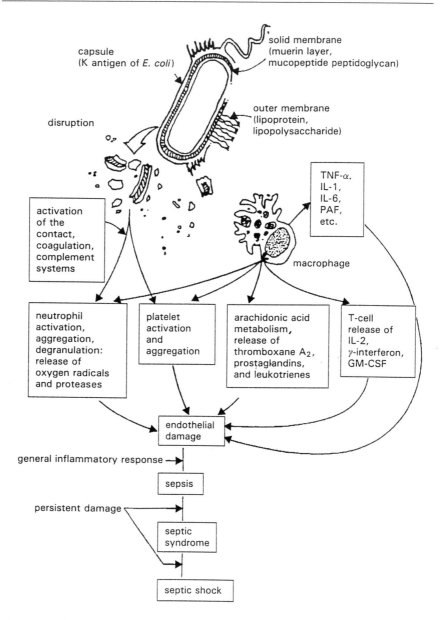

Figure 1 Schematic representation of the pathogenesis of sepsis. TNF-α, tumor necrosis factor-α; IL, interleukin; GM-CSF, granulocyte–monocyte colony-stimulating factor; PAF, platelet activating factor

25% of the adult figure. In experimental infections, the pool is depleted by 80%, compared with 33% in adults[15]. During bacterial sepsis, the daily turnover of neutrophils increases drastically and their half-life diminishes, both in animal experiments and in humans. The infection turnover in adults increases from $1.6 \times 10^{-9}\,\mathrm{PMN\,kg^{-1}day^{-1}}$ [16] to $6 \times 10^{-9}\,\mathrm{PMN\,kg^{-1}day^{-1}}$; in the neonate this implies a reserve pool depletion. In depletion due to sepsis, fewer than 7% can be present in 15% of cases[17], any moderate medullary depletion is considered a poor prognostic factor in neonatal sepsis[18], and has resulted in the development of the therapeutic granulocyte transfusion[19] and, more recently, the use of hematopoietic growth factors GM-CSF and G-CSF in animal experiments[14].

Immunoglobulins are diminished in neonates younger than 32 weeks, showing critical levels of 700–400 mg/dl[20,21] and a faster elimination rate in premature infants of very low birth weight[22]. Depending on the type of infection, there is a great variability in the range of immunoglobulin levels or utilization. From the therapeutic point of view, their efficacy in combating early infection is well documented. Further information is needed as to the mode of action of hospital-acquired infections[10], although there are antibodies[23] that give lesser protection against these bacteria, which are uncommon in the general population.

All these alterations predispose to a fatal outcome and require preventive intervention as well as an early diagnosis based on perinatal risk factors exposing the neonate to infections, hematological laboratory parameters (granulocytes – I/T (immature/total) rate, degenerative changes, medullary reserve), acute-phase reactant determinations (variable surface glycoprotein, C-reactive protein, haptoglobins, etc.) and determination of antibody levels against frequent germs and bacterial cultures[4,24,25]. If necessary, early therapeutic action should be implemented, taking into account, apart from general measures and the appropriate antibacterial therapy, the replacement of deficient immune factors, checking the damage caused by bacterial endotoxins and the pathophysiological response of the newborn during the evolution of infection, up to septic shock. If infection persists, cytokines TNF-α, IL-1 and IL-6 are released by macrophages; platelet-activating factor, arachidonic acid metabolites, eicosanoids (thromboxane A_2, leukotrienes, prostaglandin E_2, prostacyclin I_2) produced in platelets, leukocytes and macrophages, are also released. Part of the body's action is the activation of the complement and coagulation systems; all of this may imply more circulating vasoactive substances (histamine, serotonin, bradykinin) and/or consumption of coagulation factors which could lead to disseminated intravascular coagulation. On the other hand, all these factors contribute to the functional stimulation of neutrophils, with adherence to endothelial cells, lysosomal enzymes and oxidative radicals which, added to platelet aggregation, are responsible for multisystemic damage and panendothelial lesions (intravascular malignant endothelial condition)[26,27]. Knowledge of all these factors and the opportune and appropriate therapeutic intervention should improve morbidity and mortality rates during the neonatal period.

REFERENCES

1. *Departmento de Estadistica Vital Ministario de Sanidad, Asistencia Social (MSAS),* (1988–89). Venezuela
2. *Boletin informativo de su so Aniversario* (1987). Maternidad Concepción Palacios, Caracas, Venezuela
3. Yoder, M. C. and Polin, R. A. (1986). Immunotherapy of neonatal septicemia. *Ped. Clin. N. Am.*, **33**, 181–501
4. Gerdes, J. S. (1991). Clinicopathologic approach to the diagnosis of neonatal sepsis. *Clinics Perinatol.*, **19**, 961–81
5. Baker, C. J. (1991). *Immunotherapy with Intravenous Immunoglobulins,* pp. 61–74. (Academic Press)
6. Spicktt, G. P. (1992). Immune mechanisms underlying disease. *Immunol. Allergy Clinics N. Am.*, **12**, 205–12
7. Hoffbrand, A. V. and Pettit, J. E. (1988). *Clinical Haematology, Sandoz Atlas* (London, New York:Gower Medical Publishing)
8. (1986). *Ped. Inf. Dis.*, **5**(3)
9. Notarangelo, L. D., Chirico, G., Chiara, A. *et al.* (1984). Activity of classic and alternative pathways of complement in preterm and small for gestational age infants. *Ped. Res.*, **18**, 1984
10. Stanton, F. and Doran, J. E. (1991). Current status of fibronectin in transfusion medicine. Focus on Clinical Studies. *Vox Sang.*, **60**, 193–202
11. Hill, H. P. (1987). Biochemical, structural and functional abnormalities of polymorphonuclear leukocytes in the neonate. *Ped. Res.*, **22**, 375–82
12. Cairo, M. S. (1989). Review of G-CSF and GM-CSF effects on neonatal neutrophil kinetics. *Am. J. Ped. Hematol. Oncol.*, **11**(2), 238–44

13. Christiensen, R. D. (1990). Granulocytopoiesis in the fetus and neonate. *Transfusion Medicine Reviews*, **4**(1), 8–13
14. Cairo, M. S. (1992). Cytokines: a new immunotherapy. *Clin. Perinatol.*, **18**, 343–59
15. Christiensen, R. D., Macfarlane, I. L., Taylor, N. L. *et al.* (1982). Blood and marrow neutrophil during experimental group O streptococcal infection: quantification of stem cell, proliferative, storage and circulante pools. *Ped. Res.*, **16**, 549–53
16. Christiensen, R. D. (1982). Neutrophil kinetics in the fetus and neonate. *Am. J. Ped. Hematol. Oncol.*, **11**(2), 215–23
17. Engle, W. A., McGuire, W. A., Schreiner, R. L. and Yu, P.-L. (1988). Neutrophil storage pool depletion in neonates with sepsis and neutropenia. *J. Ped.*, **113**(4), 747–9
18. Cairo, M. S. (1989). Neutrophil transfusions in the treatment of neonatal sepsis. *Am. J. Ped. Hematol. Oncol.*, **11**, 227–34
19. Cairo, M. S. (1990). The use of granulocyte transfusions in neonatal sepsis. *Transfusion Medicine Reviews*, **4**, 11–22
20. Clapp, D. W., Baley, J. E. *et al.* (1989). Use of intravenously administered immune globulin to prevent nosacomial sepsis in low birth weight infants. Report of pilot study. *J. Ped.*, **115**, 973–8
21. Valbuena, A. A., Torres, M. T. *et al.* (1989). Gammaglobulina intravenosa come profilaxis de infección en el recien necido pretérmino. *Arch. Venezolanos de Farmacologia Terapéutica*, **8**, 195–201
22. Kay, S., Kyllonen, K. S., Clapp, D. W. *et al.* (1989). Dosage of intravenously administered immune globulin and dosing interval required to maintain target levels of immunoglobulin G in low birth weight infants. *J. Ped.*, **115**, 1012–16
23. Weisman, L. E., Stoll, B., Kueser, T., Rubio, T. *et al.* (1990). Intravenous immunoglobulin (IVIG) therapy in medical sepsis. *Ped. Res.*, **27**, 277A (abstract 1647–9)
24. Muller, A., Muller de M. E. *et al.* (1989). Importancia de los parametros hematológicos en el diagnostico de la infección neonatal. Uso de la gammaglobulina intravenosa. *Plasma*, **14**, 111
25. Siegel, J. D. (1990). *Sepsis Neonatorum Principles and Practice of Pediatrics*, pp. 471–9. (Lippincott)
26. Bone, R. C. (1991). The pathogenesis of sepsis. *Ann. Int. Med.*, **115**, 457–69
27. Sullivan, J. S. and Kilpatrick, L. (1992). Cytokine elevations and mortality rate in children with sepsis. *J. Ped.*, **120**, 510–15

7

Adjunctive therapy in neonatal sepsis

J. I. Santos

There are a number of factors which account for the neonate's increased risk of infection (Table 1). The host defense mechanisms of neonates are either quantitatively or qualitatively deficient, and contribute to the increased susceptibility and severity of infections in both term and preterm infants. In addition to reduced numbers of granulocytes and their progenitors, there are functional deficiencies in neonatal polymorphonuclear neutrophils (PMNs). The newborn B and T lymphocytes are hyporesponsive and exhibit delayed maturation; term newborns have low levels of IgM and IgA, and in preterm infants serum IgG levels are

Table 1 Abnormalities in host defense mechanisms in the term and preterm newborn infant

Physical barriers:	
skin and mucous membranes	deficient or compromised
Humoral immunity	
antibody	deficient IgM and IgA levels
	decreased IgG levels in preterm infants
complement	decreased levels of C3/C5 and factor B
fibronectin	decreased levels
Phagocytic cells	diminished reserves
	hematopoiesis is developmentally immature
	abnormal function
Cellular immunity	deficient T-lymphocyte activity

Table 2 Prevention of neonatal sepsis with intravenous immunoglobulin
(IVIG)

				Proven sepsis		
Author	Benefit	Blinded study	Gestational age or birth weight	IGIV	no IGIV	p
Haque	yes	no	30–37 weeks	4/100 (4%)	8/50 (16%)	0.02
Chirico	yes	no	24–34 weeks	2/43 (5%)	8/40 (20%)	0.04
Clapp	yes	yes	<2.0 kg	0/56 (0%)	7/59 (12%)	0.01
Stabile	no	no	26–34 weeks	5/46 (11%)	3/48 (6%)	0.48

low because transplacental IgG transfer occurs predominantly in the latter part of the third trimester.

Despite aggressive support measures and new and more potent antimicrobial agents, the high morbidity and mortality associated with neonatal sepsis have prompted the development and implementation of adjunctive therapeutic modalities. Among the oldest of these is the use of passive immunity for temporary protection from infectious diseases. Recent advances have permitted the modification of immune serum globulin, which can be given intravenously. Animal and human experimental and clinical data support the prophylactic use of intravenous immunoglobulins to prevent serious infections in highly selected term and preterm infants. However, therapeutic trials with these preparations have not yet demonstrated a clear benefit (Table 2).

Infected neonates often develop neutropenia, and several investigators have demonstrated that PMN transfusion may improve mortality in profoundly neutropenic septic cases. However, there is general agreement that PMN transfusion is still an experimental procedure, and should be reserved for the most critically ill infants.

Additional adjunctive therapies under study include the passive administration of fibronectin, the use of recombinant cytokines such as granulocyte–monocyte and granulocyte colony-stimulating factor (GM- and G-CSF), interferon and single nutrients. The future therapy of neonatal sepsis will probably include adjunctive immunotherapy which is predicated on our further study and under-standing of the neonate's host defense mechanisms.

METHODS

A multicenter, double-blind study was carried out of neonates weighing 500–1750 g at birth. A total of 588 neonates were randomly assigned, with stratification for birth weight, to receive periodic intravenous infusions of either immunoglobulin (500 mg/kg body weight per day) or a placebo. Mortality, morbidity and nosocomial infection were assessed during the subsequent 56 days.

RESULTS

There was a significant reduction in the risk of a first nosocomial infection in the recipients of immunoglobulin as compared to the placebo group (relative risk, 0.7; 95% confidence interval, 0.5–0.9); 85% of the nosocomial infections were bacterial, the majority of which were caused by coagulase-negative staphylococci or *Staphylococcus aureus*. The neonates who received immunoglobulin had fewer mean days of hospitalization than the controls (62 and 68, respectively; $p = 0.15$).

CONCLUSIONS

For premature infants weighing between 500 and 1750 g at birth, treatment with intravenous infusions of immunoglobulin is safe and reduces the risk of nosocomial infection.

8

Use of immunoglobulin in the treatment of burns

F. Benaim

INTRODUCTION

The action of heat in its different forms (fire, boiling or flammable fluids) or of other agents, whether physical (electricity, radiation) or chemical (different acids or caustic agents), on the skin or other tissues causes local alterations (burns) of different magnitudes, according to the intensity of the agent and the duration of its action.

Damage to the skin and/or mucous membranes by burning manifests in different forms (Table 1):

(1) As a simple reddening caused by vascular congestion (epidermic or erythematous A-type burn);

(2) By the presence of a phlyctena or blister when, in addition to congestion, there is an alteration of capillary permeability (surface dermal burn or phlyctenular A-type burn);

(3) By mortification of the epidermal layers and the outer part of the dermis, leaving some hair and nail tissue undamaged (intermediate (deep dermal) or AB-type burn); and

(4) By the necrosis of all skin strata (epidermis and dermis) causing a scab or dead tissue (deep (full thickness) burn).

Healthy skin and mucous membranes are the natural physical barriers the organism uses to defend itself from bacterial penetration from the

Table 1 Depth of burns and their description

	Description	Histological level
A-type burn (superficial)	erythematous phlyctenular	epidermis outer strata of dermis
AB-type burn	intermediate	inner strata of dermis (deep dermal)
B-type burn	deep	total skin structure (full thickness)

outside, or from blood dissemination of those within the intestinal tract. When a burn destroys that barrier, the penetration of bacteria and their reproduction prompt the body to initiate a defensive process, with the participation of all the mechanisms in the immune system. This situation is more serious when the burns are of the intermediate (AB) type, where both the epidermis and part of the dermis are destroyed, and worse still in deep burns (B type), where the whole skin structure is dead. When the process extends over certain limits (B type of more than 20% of the surface area), the lack of skin defense and the presence of necrotic tissue that originates toxic products and stimulates bacterial reproduction create a clinical condition whose severity depends on the area involved.

In these circumstances, the first defenses to be mobilized are the non-specific ones (inflammatory response), and if this barrier is overcome by the virulence of the process, specific immune systems come into action. In order to assess the real severity of the process and make a prognosis

Table 2 Severity of burn wounds according to prognosis. Severity groups or clinical forms in patients aged 12–60 years

Depth	Group I (slight)	Group II (moderate)	Group III (serious)	Group IV (critical)
A-type (superficial)	up to 10%	11–30%	31–60%	>60%
AB-type (intermediate)	up to 5%	6–15%	16–40%	>40%
B-type (deep)	up to 1%	2–5%	6–20%	>20%

on life expectancy, the extent and depth of the burns must be considered (Table 2). A practical way of expressing this in order to diagnose the clinical form or the severity group (Table 2) is to use a code, placing the total extent of the burn over a horizontal line and the partial extent corresponding to each type of burn beneath it; for example, a patient with a 60% burn, of which 20% is superficial (A), 10% is intermediate (AB) and 30% is deep (B), equivalent to a critical clinical form or group IV, will be identified as follows:

$$\frac{60}{A:20;\ AB:10;\ B:30} = IV$$

In order to diagnose the depth of the burn one can explore the degree of sensitivity, remembering that A-type burns show hyperesthesia (compression of sensitive nerve endings by local edema), AB-type burns show hypoesthesia, and B-type burns show analgesia (destruction of nerve endings).

To assess the extent of the burn, use the 'hand rule': the palm of the hand is equivalent to 1% of a person's body area.

Age and previous illness must also be taken into account because they add risk factors. Children and the elderly are more vulnerable than young people and adults, and previous or concurrent illness weakens defenses.

Garcés Salinas proposed a numerical index to assess the severity of burns, as follows:

Age
% A burn × 1
% AB burn × 2
% B burn × 3

Example: Garcés index in a 40-year-old patient with a 50% burn: 20% type A; 10% type AB; 20% type B.

Age: 40 years	Age:	40 years
	A:	20 × 1 = 20
	AB:	10 × 2 = 20
	B:	20 × 3 = $\underline{60}$

$$Burn: \frac{50}{A:20;\ AB:10;\ B:20} = IV\ index = 140$$

Sandor and Schlotterer[1] propose to add the percentage of B-type burns multiplied by 3 to the total burned area. For example, in a patient with a 60% burn, of which 5% is of the B-type, the Sandor index would be 60 + (3 × 5) = 75. Obviously, burns in groups III and IV, or serious/critical burns with a high numerical index, are more at risk and therefore the most serious.

The impact a serious or critical burn (groups III or IV) has on the organism in general is manifested in the alterations produced in the metabolic, endocrine and immune responses.

Metabolic alterations appear as hypercatabolism, which increases the metabolic rate and results in a pronounced loss of body weight, which is worsened by a lack of appetite interfering with normal food intake.

The *endocrine response* induces changes in cortisol and glucagon serum levels.

The *immune response* shows to what extent the defensive systems of the body can check the advance of bacteria and neutralize infection, which is the main cause of death in these patients.

DEFENSE MECHANISMS

The human body has a set of defensive systems which, in normal conditions, protects it from external aggression and from the action of bacteria. These are physical and chemical barriers, non-specific immune systems, and specific immune systems.

Physical barriers are the skin and mucous membranes which, when sound, prevent the invasion of surface bacteria. *Chemical defenses* are gastric acidity and the efficient secretion and excretion of defensive substances. Normal endogenous intestinal flora and peristaltic movement also contribute to maintaining the equilibrium of the organism.

The *non-specific immune system* is responsible for conditioning the inflammatory response, with the participation of circulating granulocytes (neutrophils, eosinophils), monocytes and fixed cells of the reticuloendothelial system (macrophages) mobilized by chemical mediators interleukin-1 (IL-1) and interferon (IFN). This phagocytic activity begins with leukocyte margination and then, after a process of chemotaxis, the bacteria are engulfed (phagocytosis) and later destroyed (bacteriolysis) inside the phagocytic cell. Chemotaxis is stimulated by the activated complement and by other chemoattractants, and phagocytosis is favored by opsonization.

The complement system consists of complex serum proteins that intervene in phagocytosis, neutralize viruses, regulate capillary permeability and participate in chemotaxis and opsonization. It is activated by the presence of antibodies.

The *specific immune system* is represented by T lymphocytes derived from the thymus (cell immunity), and B lymphocytes or bursa equivalents, which secrete immunoglobulin (humoral immunity). These are all activated by the presence of antigens, and this activation is regulated by stimulating cells (helper cells), suppressive agents and by the action of monocytes and macrophages. Activated T lymphocytes undergo transformation and differentiation, whereby they can exert a direct cytotoxic action, secrete lymphokines (IL-2), recruit other cells and regulate co-operation between stimulant or helper cells and suppressor cells. Activated B lymphocytes become plasma cells secreting immunoglobulin.

ALTERATIONS OF THE IMMUNE SYSTEM
CAUSED BY BURNS

The destruction of the skin barrier caused by a burn is the first step of a whole process whereby the patient's immune system will be tested.

Inhalatory lesions, frequent in burns produced inside closed rooms, produce alterations in the mucous membranes of the respiratory tract. Blood stasis and intestinal paralysis, usually observed in severe burns, alter the mucous membranes of the digestive system causing bacterial translocation, which allows intestinal bacteria to enter the bloodstream.

Endotoxins generated in the wound, plus those added by bacterial translocation, induce the production of IL-6. Their number is relative to the serum level of the endotoxin, and also reflects clinical complications.

The non-specific inflammatory response mobilizes the phagocytic system, which tries to confine the aggression.

The complement system is also altered by burns. Lower B-lymphocyte activation due to an increment in suppressor activity conditions a lower production of IgG and a subsequent diminution in complement activation. C3 and C5 fractions are diminished and, as a consequence, the whole process of opsonization, chemotaxis and phagocytosis is diminished. If the bacteria are so virulent as to overpower this line of defense, specific immune systems come into action.

In the last 30 years, many publications have addressed this subject, pointing to the different clinical and laboratory data showing the degree of such alterations.

With reference to the immune response, both humoral and cellular, the variation in IgG levels has been emphasized by a number of authors[2-5], all of whom found a decrease in values during the acute phase, a return to normal after the first week and then even a rise over normal values in some cases. This immunoglobulin level curve is only found in patients who survive; when the IgG level remains low, this is an indicator of a poor outcome.

The decrease in IgG has been considered as being due to a decreased synthesis related to an increased metabolism, increased passage into the interstitial space and loss through the exudate.

A lower rejection response to allografts is another indication of a diminished immune response, both humoral and cellular[6-8].

The reduced action of phagocytes and macrophages has been experimentally studied[9] and was demonstrated in clinical practice, as well as the deficient action of T and B lymphocytes[10].

The introduction of early tangential excision was studied[11] to assess its immunological impact on the bone marrow; it was found that there was a growth inhibition of granulocytes as well as T and B lymphocytes, together with a fall in IgG level[12]. Baar and Lawrence[13], in an experimental study on guinea pigs, found that the immunosuppressive phase characterized by the fall in IgG level was lower in animals that had undergone tangential excision on the third day, as compared to controls who had had no excision. Looking for factors responsible for immunoregulation, Voorting-Hawkin and Michael[14] found a direct relationship between the immunological changes and the serum levels of glycoproteins.

As burns cause a reduction in the number of suppressor cells, the regulation of IgE synthesis by T lymphocytes and their secretion products causes an elevation of IgE levels[15] that can be interpreted as a protective mechanism[16]. An increase in serum IgE levels has been found in patients with >20% burns. In some patients these findings have been considered to be indicators of a history of allergy[17].

In their study of immunoglobulin polyclonal production in burns patients, Teodorczyk-Injeyan and colleagues[18] believed that changes in immunoglobulin synthesis were due to deficient helper cells, rather than to a greater development of suppressors.

IMMUNOLOGICAL TREATMENT

All of these findings prompt the search for treatment that could improve immunological depression and combat infection. As early as 1964, Kefalides and co-workers[19] assessed the therapeutic action of γ-globulin associated with the use of antibiotics in the prevention of infection in severe burns. More recently, Shirani and associates[20] studied the use of modified IgG in the treatment of patients with burns, and Winkelstein[21] analyzed immunological alterations in burns, confirming the fall of IgG levels. Mono- and polyvalent vaccines[22] and intravenous immuno-globulin (IVIG) have also been used.

In a prospective randomized clinical study carried out in 20 patients who had received preventive doses of IVIG (10 patients received albumin as a control and 10 were treated with IgG), there were no statistically significant differences between the two groups, neither in the mortality rate nor in the morbidity due to sepsis, incidence of positive hemoculture, qualitative biopsies, urine culture or catheter culture. Neither was there any improvement in the chemotactic and bacteriolytic indices of neutrophils, nor in the function of lymphocytes or the relationship between suppressor and stimulant cells (helper cells)[23]. In contrast, a significant improvement was found in the incidence of polymicrobial blood cultures, cytomegalovirus titers and blood levels of endotoxins in the patients treated. The group of patients under study showed a high incidence of inhalatory lesions, so that conclusions cannot readily be drawn.

The cautious use of IVIG associated with other therapeutic agents, such as antibiotics, polymyxin B, fibronectin and immunomodulating agents, as well as good nutritional support, the early elimination of necrotic tissue and immediate skin coverage, currently constitutes the treatment of choice for patients with severe burns. The doses of IVIG to be used are 500–1000 mg/kg every 7 days. In patients undergoing excision, other doses must be added on the first postoperative day and then it must continue every 7 days.

The action of IVIG improves chemotaxis and phagocytosis, increasing opsonic activity and improving the endotoxic condition. In a group of patients clinically studied, Sica and colleagues[24] found a fall in mortality and fewer septic complications.

Fibronectin is a strong opsonizing agent that diminishes in severe burns, such diminution being relative to the degree of sepsis. When given to the patient, normal levels are regained, but there is no evidence of its action on sepsis.

Immunomodulators, such as levamisol, TP5, thymopeptins, isoprinosin, cimetidine, cyclophosphamide, metisoprinol and other drugs have been used to enhance IgG action and to produce T-lymphocyte maturity.

Transfer factor was effective in a series that was given treatment but was not randomized; immunological parameters were improved[22].

The addition of IL-2 and other mediators has produced no demonstrable clinical improvement, and prostaglandin E_2 (PGE$_2$) inhibition has little effect on the immunological response itself, since it acts on the inflammatory process.

Indomethacin inhibits the synthesis of prostaglandins and can be used intravenously, thus obtaining an improvement in cellular immunity parameters, particularly of IL-2R, but results have not been statistically significant in reducing sepsis and mortality. Combined thymopoietin and indomethacin have been effective as regards improving the immunological response in animals experimentally burned.

In order to neutralize the effect of endotoxins, monoclonal antibodies, charcoal hemofiltration and fragments of antiendotoxin Fab and polymyxin B have been used. Polymyxin B can regulate the induction of IL-6, which is a marker of infection severity[22]. Commercial IgG also has antiendotoxin activity. More recently, Magliacani and Stella[25] analyzed the use of γ-globulin and immunomodulators in the treatment of infection in severely burned patients. Thymostimulin has been used in doses of $1-1.5 \, \mathrm{mg \, kg^{-1} \, day^{-1}}$ during the first week, and then every other day up to the third or fourth week. At present, all therapeutic efforts to control sepsis and to improve the immunological condition of severely burned patients tend to check endotoxemia, stimulate cell immunity and inhibit the excess production of cyclooxygenase.

Clinical symptoms to be taken into account in the diagnosis of sepsis can be summarized by the presence of paralytic ileus after the third day, confusion, hypothermia or fever. Laboratory tests can detect an intravascular disseminated coagulopathy, and blood, urine, sputum and catheter cultures are positive. Serial quantitative biopsies are another valuable element for diagnostic and follow-up purposes, as well as determination of IgG serum levels 15 min before and 1, 24 and 96 h after infusion of IgG.

As a final summary, with reference to the use of immunoglobulin in the treatment of the severely burned patient, the following recommendations can be made:

(1) Do not use IgG routinely as prevention;

(2) Do not continue the administration of immunoglobulin for therapeutic purposes for more than 7 or 10 days, since within this period its serum level returns to normal values;

(3) Use IgG only in patients whose serum level is 300 mg/100 ml or lower;

(4) Use IgG in children as a means of protection against cytomegalovirus; and

(5) Do not disregard the positive action of the joint use of IgG and immunomodulators.

GENERAL TREATMENT

The therapeutic measures recommended above to improve the immunological response must always be accompanied by intense general treatment. In order to counteract hypercatabolism, a patient should receive a daily balanced diet that will furnish 2800 kcal/m^2 of total body area, including 20% proteins, 2% arginine, 10% lipids and 68% carbohydrates, either by mouth or via the parenteral route whenever justified. Wilmore and colleagues[26] recommend the use of α- and β-blockers as a means to diminish metabolic rate (phentolamine plus propranolol). High-protein diets maintain good serum transferrin, C3 and IgG levels and therefore they increase the opsonic index.

Specific antibiotics, used cautiously according to bacteriological studies that should guide their choice, are a good therapeutic resource. It is advisable to check their serum level to verify efficacy and to adjust the dose. It must be kept in mind that, in order to obtain a useful serum level, doses must be relative to the extent of the burn.

Early and intensive surgical treatment, eliminating burned tissue and covering the bloody areas with allografts immediately, as the case requires, is mandatory to save life in critical cases. The assistance offered by skin banks in supplying the necessary amount and quality of homografts is a valuable resource for the treatment of such patients. The use of cultured epidermis, recently incorporated into practice, is a new contribution to the achievement of autologous skin coverage, even in cases with extensive deep burns where 60–70% of the body area is affected.

The rational use of all these therapeutic measures, applied by a competent interdisciplinary group of professionals acting in an appropriate environment, offers new and promising possibilities of life to the severely burned patient[27].

REFERENCES

1. Sandor, G. and Schlotterer, M. (1978). Immunoglobulin G level, a mortality index during the hydroelectric phase of burn injury. *Burns*, **5**, 192–4
2. Arturson, G., Hogman, C. F. and Johansson, S. G. D. (1969). Changes in Ig levels in severely burned patients. *Lancet*, **1**, 546
3. Munster, A. M., Hoagland, C. and Pruit, B. A. (1970). The effect of thermal injury on serum immunoglobulins. *Ann. Surg.*, **172**, 965
4. Baar, S. (1970). Plasma protein changes in mild thermal trauma. *J. Trauma*, **19**, 684
5. Daniels, J. C., Larson, D. L. Abston, S. *et al.* (1974). Serum protein profiles in thermal burns. *J. Trauma*, **14**, 137
6. Rapaport, F. T., Converse, J. M., Horn, L. *et al.* (1964). Altered reactivity to skin homografts in severe thermal injury. *Ann. Surg.*, **159**, 390
7. Markley, K., Thornton, S. W. and Smallman, E. (1971). The effect of traumatic and non traumatic shock on allograft survival. *Surg.*, **70**, 667
8. Glaser, M. and Nelken, D. (1972). Inhibitory effect of alpha globulin on the second set allograft reaction. *Proc. Soc. Exp. Biol. Med.*, **140**, 998
9. Di Maio, A., Di Mario, D. and Jacques, L. (1976). Phagocytosis in experimental burns. *J. Surg. Res.*, **21**, 437
10. Casso, N. P. R., Gesner, B. M., Converse, J. M. *et al.* (1968). Immunosuppressive sequelae of thermal trauma. *J. Trauma*, **19**, 684

11. Janzecovic, -. (1970). A new concept in the early excision and immediate grafting of burns. *J. Trauma*, **10**, 1103
12. Asko-Seljavaara, S., Sundell, B. and Rytömaa, B. (1975). The effect of early excision on bone marrow cell growth in burned mice. *Burns*, **2**, 140
13. Baar, S. and Lawrence, J. C. (1979). The immunoglobulin response to thermal injury and tangential excision. *Burns*, **5**, 236-9
14. Voorting-Hawkin, M. and Michael, G. J. (1977). Isolation and characterization of immunoregulatory factors from normal human serum. *J. Immunol.*, **118**, 505
15. Ishizaka, K. (1984). Regulation of IgE synthesis. *Ann. Rev. Immunol.*, **2**, 159
16. Shorr, R. M., Ershler, N. B. and Gamalli, R. L. (1984). Immunoglobulin production in burned patients. *J. Trauma*, **24**, 319
17. Polacek, M., Jira, M., Fara, J., Strejcek, R. and Konigova, R. (1987). Immunoglobulin E (IgE) in patients with severe burns. *Burns*, **13**, 458-61
18. Teodorczyk-Injeyan, J. A., Sparkes, B. G., Falk, R. E. and Peters, W. J. (1986). Polyclonal immunoglobulin production in burned patients. Kinetics and correlations with T cell activity. *J. Trauma*, **26**, 834
19. Kefalides, N. A., Aranaja, B. *et al.* (1964). Evaluation of antibiotic prophylaxis and gamma-globulin, plasma, albumin and saline in severe burns. *Ann. Surg.*, **159**, 496
20. Shirani, K. Y., Vaughan, G. M., McManus, A. T. *et al.* (1984). Replacement therapy with modified immunoglobulin G in burn patients. Preliminary kinetic studies. *Am. J. Med.*, **78**, 175
21. Winkelstein, A. (1984). What are the immunological alterations induced by burn injury? *J. Trauma*, **24**, 72
22. Munster, A. M. (1987). Immunization therapy in burn patients. In Baswick, J. A. Jr. (ed.) *The Art and Science of Burn Care*. (Rockville, MD:Aspen Publications)
23. Munster, A. M., Moran, K. T., Thupari, J., Allo, M. and Winchurch, R. A. (1987). Prophylactic intravenous immunoglobulin replacement in high-risk burn patients. *J.B.C.R.*, **8**, 376
24. Sica, I., Gonzalez Oliva, R., Goenaga, C. and Filipini, C. (1985). Utilizacion de la Immunoglobulina endovenosa en los quemados graves. *Rev. Arg. Quem.*, **3**
25. Magliacani, C. and Stella, M. (1990). The use of gammaglobulins and immunomodulators in the therapy of infections in serious burn patients. *Ann. Mediterranean Burns Club*, **3**, 8
26. Wilmore, -. *et al.* (1974). *Ann. Surg.*, **180**, 653
27. Benaim, F. (1992). Avances y nuevos horizontes en el tratamiento de las quemaduras. *La Prensa Med. Arg.*, **79**, 8

9

Variable region–dependent regulation of autoreactivity by intravenous immunoglobulin

V. Ruiz de Souza, M. D. Kazatchkine and S. V. Kaveri

Therapeutic preparations of normal immunoglobulin for intravenous use (IVIG) are obtained from the plasma of a large number of healthy blood donors. Most IVIG preparations that are now available contain more than 95% intact IgG, with a subclass distribution similar to that of IgG in normal serum, a half-life of 3 weeks *in vivo* and an antibody content that represents the wide spectrum of expressed antibody activities in normal human serum. These reactivities include antibodies to external antigens, natural antibodies to self antigens and anti-idiotypic antibodies[1,2].

IVIG was initially used as a replacement therapy in primary immunodeficiencies and as prophylactic therapy for systemic infections. In recent years, IVIG has also successfully been used in the treatment of autoimmune and systemic inflammatory diseases[3]. This review will focus on the mechanisms by which immunoglobulin may modulate expression of autoimmunity.

IVIG THERAPY IN AUTOIMMUNE AND SYSTEMIC INFLAMMATORY DISEASES

Short-term and long-term beneficial effects

The clinical use of IVIG therapy in autoimmune diseases has been reviewed in detail elsewhere[2-4]. Table 1 lists the autoimmune and

Table 1 Autoimmune and systemic inflammatory diseases in which intravenous immunoglobulin therapy is of proven or probable benefit*

Idiopathic thrombocytopenic purpura
Autoimmune hemolytic anemias
Autoimmune neutropenia

Anti-factor VIII autoimmune disease
Autoimmune erythroblastopenia
Myasthenia gravis
Guillain–Barré syndrome
Chronic inflammatory demyelinating polyneuropathy
Monoclonal gammopathies with anti-MAG activity
ANCA-positive systemic vasculitis
Systemic lupus erythematosus
Anticardiolipin antibodies and recurrent abortions
Antibodies to von Willebrand factor
Juvenile rheumatoid arthritis
Thyroid-related eye disease
Bullous pemphigoid

Birdshot retinopathy
Juvenile diabetes
Multiple sclerosis

Kawasaki disease
Refractory polymyositis
Sjögren's syndrome
Felty's syndrome
Ulcerative colitis
Crohn's disease

Graft versus host disease

*Diseases in which a clinical improvement and/or decrease in autoantibody titer has been established in clinical trials or suggested by open trials or preliminary reports; MAG, myelin-associated glycoprotein; ANCA, antineutrophil cytoplasm antibodies

systemic inflammatory diseases in which controlled or open trials have shown that IVIG therapy has resulted in clinical improvement and/or a decrease in autoantibody titers. Autoimmune diseases in which a beneficial effect of IVIG has been reported include diseases that are mediated or suggested to be mediated by autoantibodies, and diseases believed to be primarily mediated by autoaggressive T cells.

The beneficial effects of IVIG infusion have also been observed across species barriers. Thus, five daily consecutive infusions of IVIG were effective in preventing autoimmune disease in S-antigen-induced experimental autoimmune uveoretinitis, a T-cell-mediated disease occurring in susceptible strains of rats[5]. Infusion of IVIG has resulted in decreased proteinuria and suppression of increased IgE production in $HgCl_2$-induced autoimmune disease of Brown Norway rats[6]. Infusion of IVIG has also been shown to inhibit or delay the onset of experimental autoimmune arthritis induced in Lewis rats by the injection of *Mycobacterium tuberculosis* in complete Freund's adjuvant[7].

Several mechanisms of action have been proposed to explain the immunoregulatory effects of IVIG in autoimmune diseases[3,8,9]. Short-term effects of IVIG observed within days of administration may depend on one or several non-mutually exclusive mechanisms, including the neutralization of autoantibody activity through V region-dependent interactions between the patient's autoantibodies and infused IVIG, transient blockade of Fc-receptor function on fixed phagocytes,

Table 2 Possible mechanisms involved in the short-term effects of intravenous immunoglobulin in autoimmune and systemic inflammatory diseases

---

Fc-dependent mechanisms

Transient functional blockade of Fcγ receptors on phagocytic cells

Modulation of the synthesis and release of interleukins and inflammatory mediators by monocyte/macrophages

Inhibition of the binding of complement components to targets of complement activation

Changes in the structure and solubility of immune complexes

V region-dependent mechanisms

Neutralization/removal of a putative toxin, pathogen or antigen involved in pathogenesis

Neutralization of autoantibody activity through idiotypic interactions between the patient's autoantibodies and complementary antibodies in intravenous immunoglobulin

---

preventing the accelerated clearance of cells opsonized with autoantibodies, and the inhibition of release of proinflammatory monocytic cytokines (Table 2). In several autoimmune diseases, IVIG has also been shown to control autoimmune manifestations for prolonged periods of time far beyond the half-life of infused immunoglobulin; the long-term effects of IVIG therapy imply activation or down-regulation of T- and/or B-cell clones in the patient, resulting in the re-establishment of serological and cellular parameters that characterize the normal function of the immune system in healthy individuals. We have thus proposed that most of the beneficial effects (both short- and long-term) of IVIG in autoimmune patients depend on the ability of variable regions of pooled, polyspecific immunoglobulin from healthy donors to modulate expressed immune repertoires, and to restore the steady-state equilibrium of the immune system that controls the expression of autoreactivity under physiological conditions (Table 3). This ability relies on the very nature of immunoglobulins as components of the immune system actively selecting preimmune repertoires in healthy individuals, and on the diversity of V regions of IVIG as being representative of the various immunoglobulins involved in the maintenance of the homeostasis of the normal immune system. A predominant role for V region-dependent mechanisms of action of IVIG implies that the response to therapy may vary between patients. Some of the major mechanisms involved in the short-term effects of IVIG are illustrated by the diseases briefly discussed below. Emphasis will be laid on the role of V region-dependent immunoregulatory effects of IVIG, with regard to both the short- and the long-term consequences of IVIG therapy.

Table 3 V region-dependent modulation of autoimmunity by intravenous immunoglobulin (IVIG)

Short-term effects: neutralization of autoantibodies by passively transferred anti-idiotypes in IVIG

Long-term effects: V region-mediated selection of immune repertoires through activation or down-regulation of IVIG-reactive B- and/or T-cell clones

---

Blockade of Fcγ receptor by IVIG

The short-term effects of IVIG in idiopathic thrombocytopenic purpura (ITP) have been attributed to a transient blockade of Fc receptors on splenic macrophages, resulting in the decreased clearance of antibody-coated platelets[10-12]. Evidence for Fc-receptor blockade came from the finding of a decreased clearance of autologous erythrocytes coated with anti-Rh-D antibodies for about 4 weeks following treatment with IVIG[11]. Platelet survival is prolonged in ITP patients treated with IVIG. In addition, peripheral blood monocytes from IVIG-treated patients exhibit a decreased ability to form rosettes with IgG-coated erythrocytes *in vitro*[13]. Blockade of Fc receptors on macrophages following treatment of Rh-D-positive ITP patients with anti-D antibodies[12], or treatment with a monoclonal antibody directed against FcγRIII[10], mimicked the effect of IVIG by inhibiting the accelerated splenic clearance of antibody-coated platelets.

Other mechanisms of action of IVIG may, however, also operate in ITP (*see* Chapter 12), since a decreased Fc receptor-mediated clearance is not observed in all patients who respond to IVIG, and since IVIG may be effective in splenectomized patients. The interaction of IVIG with anti-GPIIb/IIIa antibodies[14] could thus contribute to the short-term effects of the treatment through the anti-idiotypic neutralization of antiplatelet autoantibodies. The long-term decrease in antiplatelet antibody production that is sometimes observed, and the re-establishment of suppressor T-cell function following IVIG therapy, indicates that IVIG also induces modifications of B- and T-cell repertoires in patients with ITP[15,16].

Modulation by IVIG of the release and the function of proinflammatory cytokines

Inhibition of the release of monocytic cytokines by IVIG may play an important role in the rapid anti-inflammatory effects of IVIG in Kawasaki syndrome. The resolution of fever is frequently apparent within a few hours of initiation of infusion. Controlled clinical trials have demonstrated that IVIG therapy reduces early inflammatory symptoms, but also significantly decreases the incidence of coronary artery abnormalities upon long-term follow-up of treated patients[17,18]. The acute vasculitic phase of Kawasaki syndrome is associated with high serum levels of interleukin-1 (IL-1), IL-6, tumor necrosis factor (TNF) and of T-cell cytokines such as γ-interferon (γ-IFN)[18], with the occurrence of antineutrophil cytoplasm antibodies (ANCA)[19] and of antibodies able to lyse cytokine-stimulated endothelial cells[20]. IVIG has been shown to inhibit the release of IL-1 and TNF from lipopolysaccharide (LPS)-activated monocytes *in vitro* (Carreno, unpublished results), and has recently been shown to stimulate the release of the natural IL-1 inhibitor, IL-1 Ra, from monocytes (Dinarello, personal communication). In experimental animals, IVIG was shown to induce an increase in cellular cyclic adenosine monophosphate (cAMP) levels in peritoneal exudate cells, which results in an inhibition of IL-1 and TNF-α production. This effect was mediated by the Fc portion of IVIG[21]. Another way in which IVIG may inhibit the functions of inflammatory cytokines is through binding to the cytokines of natural anticytokine antibodies present in IVIG. Thus, antibodies to IL-1α[22] and to IFNs are present in normal human serum[23], and anti-IL-1 antibodies have been found in IVIG[24]. The protective effect of IVIG on coronary artery damage in Kawasaki syndrome could thus be related to the decreased release and function of monocytic cytokines, decreased mononuclear cell infiltration and decreased antibody-mediated cell lysis. In this regard, it may be that anti-idiotypic modulation of antiendothelial cell antibodies plays a role in avoiding antibody-mediated vascular damage, as has been described in ANCA-positive systemic vasculitis[25].

Idiotypic neutralization of autoantibodies by IVIG

V region-dependent interactions between IVIG and disease-associated autoantibodies may account for the early decrease in autoantibody titers that have been observed in patients treated with IVIG, as has initially been described in patients with anti-factor VIII autoantibodies[26]. Inhibition of anti-factor VIII activity *in vivo* was correlated with the ability of IVIG and F(ab')$_2$ fragments of IVIG to neutralize patients' anti-factor VIII autoantibodies *in vitro*[26,27]. Neutralization of antibody activity was mediated by idiotypic interactions between anti-factor VIII autoantibodies and IVIG as demonstrated by the retention of specific anti-factor VIII autoantibody activity on affinity columns of sepharose-bound F(ab')$_2$ fragments of IVIG[27,28] and the ability of IVIG to compete for the binding to an anti-factor VIII autoantibody of a murine monoclonal antibody directed against a paratope-related idiotope of anti–factor VIII antibodies[29]. As discussed below, idiotypic interactions between autoantibodies and anti–idiotypes in IVIG are not only critical to the short-term effects of IVIG, but also important in determining the interactions between IVIG and lymphocytes that may lead to the long-term suppression of autoantibody–secreting clones in treated patients.

VARIABLE REGION-DEPENDENT LONG-TERM REGULATION OF AUTOREACTIVITY BY IVIG

Network control of autoreactivity in healthy individuals

Natural autoantibodies of the IgM and IgG isotypes are present in the serum of healthy individuals[30]. These antibodies recognize a wide panel of autoantigens, including cell surface components (e.g. acetylcholine receptors, idiotypes of antigen receptors), intracellular molecules (e.g. DNA) and extracellular molecules (e.g. insulin and intrinsic factor)[31-33]. Some of the autoantigens recognized by the natural autoantibodies are targets of autoantibodies in autoimmune disease. Natural autoantibodies are often polyreactive. Under physiological conditions, the available (selected) B-cell repertoire and the expressed autoreactive repertoire (i.e. natural autoantibodies) are controlled within a network of V region-dependent interactions.

Physiological autoreactivity is now recognized as a feature of the normal immune system that is required for the establishment and maintenance of repertoires in the healthy individual[34]. Studies in mice and humans have shown that the predominantly selected repertoire in the neonate is self-reactive and multispecific[35], and that it favors the use of certain viral hepatitis gene families[36] (F. Huetz and colleagues, unpublished observations). It is then driven by epigenetic processes involving maternal antibodies[37,38], autologous B and T cells and idiotypes of immunoglobulins[39-41] as well as antigens. Although there are differences in the usage of viral hepatitis genes and somatic diversity between neonatal and adult repertoires, physiological autoreactivity persists in the adult and is maintained in the pool of naturally activated lymphocytes. The selection and maintenance of this normal autoreactive repertoire is a recursive process dependent on V region-dependent interactions that establish connectivity between antibodies and cells in the normal immune system[42,43]. Pathological autoimmunity is associated with a loss or decrease in connectivity that allows the abnormal expansion of autoreactive clones.

Direct evidence for intrinsic network regulation of the autoreactive B-cell repertoire in healthy adults comes from the observation of reproducible patterns of spontaneous kinetic behavior of natural autoantibodies in serum. These patterns are similar to those observed in normal mice, and reflect the regulation of activation and decay of autoantibody clones within a network organization. In contrast, autoantibodies in the serum of patients with autoimmune disease follow random spontaneous fluctuations suggestive of an acquired loss of control of the expressed autoreactive repertoire. The abnormal kinetic behavior of autoantibodies in autoimmune patients affects disease-associated autoantibodies as well as natural autoantibodies that are not directly involved in the pathological process. Thus, autoimmune disease appears to be associated with a general disturbance of the self-referential network, rather than with the clonally localized escape of tissue-specific autoantibodies. Recent evidence from our laboratory indicates that the infusion of IVIG in autoimmune patients switches the kinetic pattern of spontaneous autoantibody fluctuations from random to a pattern characteristic of healthy individuals (see below).

Idiotypic interactions between antibodies control expression of the autoreactive repertoire in normal human serum

V region-dependent regulation of the expressed autoreactive B-cell repertoire is apparent from the finding of a high V region connectivity among natural autoantibodies and that of V region-mediated inhibition of IgG autoreactivity by autologous IgM in normal serum. We have observed that there exists a fraction of normal circulating IgG which exhibits V region complementarity associated with autoreactivity[44]. This 'connected fraction' represents up to 0.7–1.0% of IgG in IVIG pools. Within the connected fraction of IgG are self-binding antibodies that react with their own variable region determinants. The finding of V region-dependent complementarity between autologous IgG and IgM in mice[45] and humans[46] came from the observation of a low expression of natural IgG autoantibodies in whole serum, contrasting with high titers of IgG autoantibodies in the purified IgG fraction from the serum (Figure 1). Isolated IgG from normal human serum reacts with a large panel of self-antigens, including

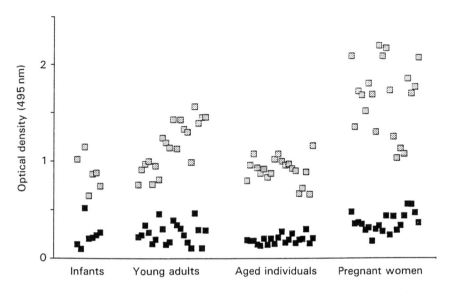

Figure 1 Comparison between the mean binding activity of purified IgG (▨) and of IgG in whole serum (■) of infants, young adults, elderly donors and pregnant women against ten autoantigens

thyroglobulin, DNA, evolutionarily conserved cytoskeletal proteins, factor VIII and intrinsic factor. No difference in autoreactivity within the purified fraction from serum was found between aged individuals, young adults and infants. The reactivity of purified IgG with autoantigens was higher for IgG from the serum of pregnant women in the last trimester of pregnancy. The addition of purified IgM to autologous IgG resulted in dose-dependent inhibition of IgG autoreactivity; inhibition was mediated by V region interactions between IgM and autologous IgG[46].

These results emphasize the role of connectivity in controlling the expression of the autoreactive repertoire in whole serum, and offers support for the therapeutic modulation of autoimmunity using intravenously administered IgM.

Idiotypic interactions between IVIG and natural or pathological antibodies

As mentioned previously, IVIG contains antibodies that recognize idiotypes expressed by disease-associated autoantibodies. Such V region-dependent interactions provide a basis for the neutralization of circulating autoantibodies in the early phase of IVIG therapy. Four lines of evidence demonstrated idiotypic interactions between IVIG and disease-associated autoantibodies:

(1) F(ab')$_2$ fragments of IVIG neutralize the functional activity of autoantibodies and/or inhibit the binding of autoantibodies to autoantigens. Inhibition of autoantibody activity has been observed in the case of anti–factor VIII autoantibodies, anti–DNA antibodies from patients with systemic lupus erythematosus (SLE), antithyroglobulin autoantibodies from patients with Hashimoto's thyroid disease, anti–intrinsic factor antibodies from patients with megaloblastic anemia, antineutrophil cytoplasmic antigen antibodies from patients with systemic vasculitis, antiperipheral nerve antibodies from patients with Guillain–Barré syndrome and chronic inflammatory demyelinating neuropathy, antiendothelial cell antibodies from patients with SLE, antierythroblast antibodies from patients with autoimmune erythroblastopenia, and antiretinal S-antigen of patients with autoimmune uveitis[27,47–49] (D. Jobin; N. Ronda and colleagues, unpublished observations).

(2) Autoantibodies specifically bind to affinity chromatography columns of F(ab')$_2$ fragments of IVIG coupled to sepharose.

(3) IVIG does not contain antiallotypic antibodies against F(ab')$_2$ regions of normal human IgG[27].

(4) IVIG shares anti–idiotypic reactivity towards idiotypes of auto-antibodies with heterologous anti–idiotypic reagents[29,50].

We have also demonstrated that IVIG interacts with natural poly-reactive IgM antibodies through V region-dependent interactions, by using autoreactive monoclonal IgM antibodies secreted by Epstein–Barr virus (EBV)-transformed normal B lymphocytes[33]. The presence in IVIG of anti-idiotypes against idiotypic determinants expressed on natural autoantibodies of the IgG isotype was demonstrated by using affinity chromatography of F(ab')$_2$ fragments of IVIG on sepharose-bound F(ab')$_2$ fragments of IVIG[44]. In addition, recent studies have shown that IVIG interacts idiotypically with complementarity-determining regions and the framework constant regions of the β chain of the human T-cell receptor[51] and with the complementarity-determining region 2/framework region 3 of murine myeloma protein

Table 4 Antilymphocyte antibodies in intravenous immunoglobulin

Antibodies to idiotypes/variable regions of surface immunoglobulin of B cells
Antibodies to idiotype, framework and constant regions of T-cell receptor
  β chain
Antibodies to CD4
Antibodies to CD5
Antibodies to major histocompatibility complex class I and class II antigens

S107/T15[52]. IVIG may thus also modulate the functions of T and B lymphocytes by interacting with cell surface molecules such as CD5, CD4 or major histocompatibility complex products[53] (V. Hurez and co-workers unpublished observations) (Table 4).

Sources of anti–idiotypic activity against autoantibodies in IVIG

Several factors may contribute to the presence in IVIG of enriched anti–idiotypic activity against autoantibodies (Table 5). Healthy, aged individuals may potentially represent a 'privileged' source of donors for anti–idiotypes in IVIG. Thus, we have recently found that IgG in the serum of donors between 50 and 60 years of age was more effective than IgG in the serum of donors between 20 and 30 years of age in inhibiting anti–factor VIII autoantibody activity[1]. A second source of anti-idiotypes may be the presence in IVIG pool of IgG from individuals having spontaneously recovered from autoimmune diseases. Analysis of the serum of patients who spontaneously recovered from anti–factor VIII autoimmune disease[28] and from other autoimmune diseases such as

Table 5 Sources of anti–idiotypic activity against autoantibodies in intravenous immunoglobulin (IVIG)

Donors with 'high' titers of anti–idiotypes against autoantibodies:
  aged donors
  pregnant/multiparous women
  individuals having spontaneously recovered from autoimmune
    diseases
Synergistic effect of pooling immunoglobulin from multiple donors
V region 'connected' fraction of IVIG

SLE[54], myasthenia gravis[55] or Guillain–Barré syndrome[49] suggested that the appearance of anti-idiotypic antibodies to acute-phase autoantibodies is associated with recovery.

Another factor accounting for the presence of an increased anti-idiotypic activity in IVIG against autoantibodies is the synergistic effect obtained from the complementation of individual antibody sources in the IVIG pool. Thus, combining IgG from three or four individuals whose IgG, when tested individually, does not express anti-idiotypic activity, results in the expression in the pool of an anti-idiotypic activity against anti-factor VIII autoantibodies[1]. As the number of donors increases, the probability of finding anti-idiotypic antibodies directed against an auto-antibody of a given idiotypic specificity increases considerably in the pool.

Selection of immune repertoires and changes in network organization induced by IVIG in autoimmune patients

Ontogenic studies using strains of mice prone to autoimmunity indicate that autoimmune disease results from the aberrant development of the immune system, leading to defective connectivity in adult animals. In the non-obese diabetic (NOD) mouse strain, which develops autoimmune diabetes (type I) after 13 weeks of age, *in situ* hybridization studies demonstrated that adult mice display abnormally the neonatal pattern of viral hepatitis gene utilization (K. Leijon and D. Holmberg, unpublished observations). Interestingly, the treatment of newborn NOD mice with natural monoclonal antibodies obtained from a non-autoimmunity-prone strain not only prevents the development of diabetes but partially restores the normal viral hepatitis gene utilization pattern (A. Andersson and colleagues, unpublished observations). The infusion of pooled mouse immunoglobulins in pathogen-free mice is efficient in selecting B-cell repertoires expressing the viral hepatitis gene families used in normal conventional adult mice, and not in germ-free mice[56].

The effect of pooled normal murine immunoglobulin has been studied in normal BALB/c mice[57]. The results show that high doses of immunoglobulin induce an increase in activated B and CD4+ T cells in the spleen, with an increase in IgM and IgG-secreting cells on the 8th day after treatment. In contrast, analysis of the bone marrow revealed a reduction in pre-B cells, suggesting a negative feedback control in B-cell differentiation mediated by V regions of isologous immunoglobulin[58].

Taken together, these results suggest that the administration of high doses of immunoglobulins results in immunostimulatory effects that could be responsible for changes in expressed repertoire. Furthermore, isologous immunoglobulins as natural components of the immune system also provide physiological signals capable of maintaining homeostasis.

We have recently analyzed the changes that occur in the expressed autoreactive antibody repertoire and in network organization following the infusion of normal polyspecific IgG in a patient with autoimmune thyroiditis[59]. The results have allowed us to gather several lines of evidence indicating that changes in serum antibody concentrations observed after infusion of IVIG do not merely reflect passive transfer of IgG into the patient. The concentration of IgG in the patient's serum after the second infusion of IVIG increased to higher levels than would be expected from the amount of transfused IgG. Accordingly, the two consecutive infusions of IVIG resulted in a cumulative increase in the production of IgM. These observations illustrate an *in vivo* activation of lymphocytes following infusion with normal immunoglobulins (Table 6).

Table 6 Selection of immune repertoires by intravenous immunoglobulin (IVIG)

Long-term suppression of disease-related B-cell clones

Restricted stimulation of B-cell clones (i.e. clones interacting through V regions with IVIG)

Altered kinetic pattern of spontaneous fluctuations of natural autoantibodies in serum, indicative of induced alterations in network organization

---

In addition, the dynamic behavior of autoantibodies in the patient prior to the infusion of immunoglobulin exhibits a clearly distinct pattern, with marked rhythmicity suggestive of disruptions of connectivity within the immune network (Figure 2). The kinetic pattern following the second infusion of IVIG, on the other hand, is similar to that seen in healthy individuals. Thus, infusion of pooled normal immunoglobulin restored in the patient a network organization of autoantibodies characteristic of the physiological conditions. These observations support our hypothesis that the beneficial effect of IVIG in autoimmune diseases is not merely due to the passive transfer (transfusion) of neutralizing anti-idiotypic

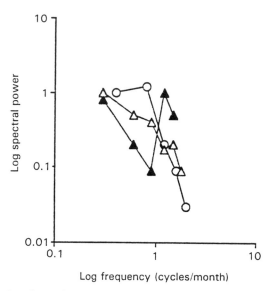

Figure 2 Spectral analysis of the fluctuations of anti-thyroglobulin autoantibodies in serum of a healthy individual (○), of a patient with Hashimoto's thyroiditis before infusion of intravenous immunoglobulin (IVIG) (▲), and following the two infusions of IVIG (△). Spectral values have been normalized

antibodies against autoantibodies, but that IVIG alters the structure and the dynamics of the idiotypic network in the autoimmune patient, so as to regain physiological control of autoimmunity (Table 6). IVIG would thus clearly differ in its mode of action from the immunosuppressive approach to the treatment of autoimmune diseases[44,60].

ACKNOWLEDGEMENTS

This work was supported by Institut National de la Santé et de la Recherche Médicale (INSERM), Centre National de la Recherche Scientifique (CNRS) France, Sandoz SA and the Central Laboratory of the Swiss Red Cross, Switzerland. V. Ruiz de Souza is a recipient of a doctoral fellowship from Conselho National de Desenvolvimento Científico e Tecnológico (CNPq), Brazil.

REFERENCES

1. Dietrich, G., Algiman, M., Sultan, Y., Nydegger, U. E. and Kazatchkine, M. D. (1992). Origin of anti-idiotypic activity against anti-factor VIII

autoantibodies in pools of normal human immunoglobulin G (IVIG). *Blood*, **79**, 2946–51

2. Rossi, F., Dietrich, G. and Kazatchkine, M. D. (1989). Anti-idiotypes against autoantibodies in normal immunoglobulins: evidence for network regulation of human autoimmune responses. *Immunol. Rev.*, **110**, 135–49

3. Dwyer, J. M. (1992). Manipulating the immune system with immune globulin. *N. Engl. J. Med.*, **326**, 107–16

4. Schwartz, S. A. (1990). Intravenous immunoglobulin (IVIg) for the therapy of autoimmune disorders. *J. Clin. Immunol.*, **10**, 81

5. Saoudi, A., Hurez, V., Kozak, Y. D., Kuhn, J., Kaveri, S. V., Kazatchkine, M. D., Druet, P. and Bellon, B. (1993). Human immunoglobulin preparations for intravenous use (IVIg) prevent experimental autoimmune uveoretinitis. Evidence for induction of anergy. *Int. Immunol.*, in press

6. Rossi, F., Bellon, B., Vial, M. C., Druet, P. and Kazatchkine, M. D. (1991). Beneficial effect of human therapeutic intravenous immunoglobulins (IVIg) in HgCl$_2$-induced autoimmune disease of Brown Norway rats. *Clin. Exp. Immunol.*, **84**, 129–33

7. Achiron, A., Margalit, R., Hershkoviz, R., Markovits, D., Lider, O. and Cohen, I. R. (1992). Suppression of adjuvant arthritis by intravenously administered immunoglobulins. *8th International Congress of Immunology*, Budapest, Hungary, August 23–28. Abstract number W90-2

8. Kaveri, S. V., Dietrich, G., Hurez, V. and Kazatchkine, M. D. (1991). Intravenous immunoglobulins (IVIg) in the treatment of autoimmune disease. *Clin. Exp. Immunol.*, **86**, 192–8

9. Ronda, N., Hurez, V. and Kazatchkine, M. D. (1992). Intravenous immunoglobulin (IVIG) therapy of autoimmune and inflammatory diseases. *Vox Sang.*, **64**, 65–72

10. Clarkson, S. B., Bussel, J. B., Kimberly, R. P., Valinsky, J. E., Nachman, R. L. and Unkeless, J. C. (1986). Treatment of refractory immune thrombocytopenic purpura with an anti-Fc γ-receptor antibody. *N. Engl. J. Med.*, **314**, 1236–9

11. Fehr, J., Hofmann, V. and Kappeler, U. (1982). Transient reversal of thrombocytopenia in idiopathic thrombocytopenic purpura by high-dose intravenous gammaglobulin. *N. Engl. J. Med.*, **306**, 1254–8

12. Salama, A., Mueller-Eckhardt, C. and Kiefel, V. (1983). Effect of intravenous immunoglobulin in immune thrombocytopenia. Competitive inhibition of reticuloendothelial system function by sequestration of autologous red blood cells? *Lancet*, **2**, 193–5

13. Kimberly, R. P., Salmon, J. E., Bussel, J. B., Kuntz, Crow, M. and Hilgartner, M. W. (1984). Modulation of mononuclear phagocyte function by intravenous γ-globulin. *J. Immunol.*, **132**, 745–50

14. Berchtold, P., Dale, G. L., Tani, P. and McMillan, R. (1989). Inhibition of autoantibody binding to platelet glycoprotein IIb/IIIa by anti-idiotypic antibodies in intravenous immunoglobulins. *Blood*, **74**, 2414–17

15. Bussel, J. B., Kimberly, R. P., Inman, R. D., Schulman, I., Cunningham-Rundles, C., Cheung, N., Smithwick, M., O'Malley, J., Barandum, S. and Hilgartner, H. W. (1983). Intravenous γ-globulin treatment of chronic idiopathic thrombocytopenic purpura. *Blood*, **62**, 480–6

16. Delfraissy, J. F., Tchernia, G., Laurian, Y., Wallon, C. and Galanaud, P. (1985). Suppressor cell function after intravenous γ-globulin treatment in adult chronic idiopathic thrombocytopenic purpura. *Br. J. Haematol.*, **60**, 315–22

17. Newburger, J. W., Takahashi, M., Burns, J. C., Beiser, A. S., Chung, K. J., Duffy, C. E., Glode, M. P., Mason, W. H., Reddy, V., Sanders, R. P., Shulman, S. T., Wiggins, J. W., Hicks, R. V., Fulton, D. R., Lewis, A. B., Leung, D. Y. M., Colton, T., Rosen, F. S. and Melish, M. E. (1986). The treatment of Kawasaki syndrome with intravenous γ-globulin. *N. Engl. J. Med.*, **315**, 341

18. Rowley, A. H., Gonzalez-Crussi, F. and Shulman, S. T. (1991). Kawasaki Syndrome. *Curr. Probl. Pediatr.*, **21**, 387–405

19. Savage, C. O. S., Tizard, J. and Jayne, D. R. W. (1989). Anti-neutrophil cytoplasm antibodies in Kawasaki disease. *Arch. Dis. Child.*, **64**, 360–3

20. Leung, D. Y. M., Geha, R. S. and Newburger, J. W. (1986). Two monokines, interleukin 1 and tumor necrosis factor, render cultured vascular endothelial cells susceptible to lysis by antibodies circulating during Kawasaki Syndrome. *J. Exp. Med.*, **164**, 1958–72

21. Shimozato, T., Iwata, M., Kawada, H. and Tamura, N. (1991). Human immunoglobulin preparation for intravenous use induces elevation of cellular cyclic adenosine 3′: 5′-monophosphate levels, resulting in suppression of tumor necrosis factor α and interleukin-1 production. *Immunology*, **72**, 497–501

22. Saurat, J. H., Schifferli, J. A., Steiger, G., Dayer, J. M. and Didierjean, L. (1991). Anti-interleukin 1-α autoantibodies in humans: characterization, isotype distribution, and receptor binding inhibition – higher frequency in Schnitzler's syndrome. *J. Allergy Clin. Immunol.*, **88**, 244–56

23. Ross, C., Hansen, M. B., Schyberg, T. and Berg, K. (1990). Autoantibodies to crude human leucocyte interferon (IFN), native human IFN, recombinant human IFN-α-2b and human IFN-γ in healthy blood donors. *Clin. Exp. Immunol.*, **82**, 57–62

24. Schifferli, J. A., Saurat, J. H. and Didierjean, L. (1991). Immunomodulatory effects of intravenous immunoglobulin G. *J. Rheumatol.*, **18**, 937–9

25. Jayne, D. R. W., Davies, M., Fox, C. and Lockwood, C. M. (1991). Treatment of systemic vasculitis with pooled intravenous immunoglobulin. *Lancet*, **2**, 1137–9

26. Sultan, Y., Kazatchkine, M. D., Maisonneuve, P. and Nydegger, U. (1984). Anti-idiotypic suppression of autoantibodies to Factor VIII (anti-haemophilic factor) by high-dose intravenous gammaglobulin. *Lancet*, **2**, 765–8

27. Rossi, F., Sultan, Y. and Kazatchkine, M. D. (1988). Anti-idiotypes against autoantibodies and alloantibodies to Factor VIIIc (anti-hemophilic factor) are present in therapeutic polyspecific normal immunoglobulins. *Clin. Exp. Immunol.*, **74**, 311–16

28. Sultan, Y., Rossi, F. and Kazatchkine, M. D. (1987). Recovery from anti-VIIIc (anti-hemophilic factor) autoimmune disease is dependent on generation of anti-idiotypes against anti-VIIIc autoantibodies. *Proc. Natl. Acad. Sci. USA*, **84**, 828–31

29. Dietrich, G., Pereira, P., Algiman, M., Sultan, Y. and Kazatchkine, M. D. (1990). A monoclonal anti-idiotypic antibody against the antigen-combining site of anti-factor VIII autoantibodies defines an idiotope that is recognized by normal human polyspecific immunoglobulins for therapeutic use (IVIg). *J. Autoimmun.*, **3**, 547–57

30. Dietrich, G. and Kazatchkine, M. D. (1992). Human natural self-reactive antibodies. In Coutinho, A. and Kazatchkine, M. D. (eds.) *Autoimmunity Today*. (New York: John Wiley & Sons)

31. Avrameas, S., Guilbert, B. and Dighiero, G. (1981). Natural antibodies against tubulin, actin, myoglobin, thyroglobulin, fetuin, albumin and transferrin are present in normal human sera and monoclonal immunoglobulins from multiple myeloma and Waldenström's macroglobulinemia may express similar antibody specificities. *Ann. Immunol.* (Inst. Pasteur), **132C**, 231–6

32. Prabhakar, B. S., Saegusa, J., Onodera, T. and Notkins, A. L. (1984). Lymphocytes capable of making monoclonal antibodies that react with multiple organs are a common feature of the normal B cell repertoire. *J. Immunol.*, **133**, 2815–17

33. Rossi, F., Guilbert, B., Tonnelle, C., Ternynck, T., Fumoux, F., Avrameas, S. and Kazatchkine, M. D. (1990). Idiotypic interactions between normal human polyspecific IgG and natural IgM antibodies. *Eur. J. Immunol.*, **20**, 2089–94

34. Holmberg, D. and Kearney, J. F. (1992). Selection of the B cell repertoire and natural autoantibodies. In Coutinho, A. and Kazatchkine, M. D. (eds.) *Autoimmunity Today*. (New York: John Wiley & Sons)

35. Holmberg, D., Forsgren, S., Ivars, F. and Coutinho, A. (1984). Reactions amongst IgM antibodies derived from normal, neonatal mice. *Eur. J. Immunol.*, **14**, 435–41

36. Alt, F., Yancopoulos, G. D., Blackwell, T. K., Wood, C., Thomas, E., Boss, M., Coffman, R., Rosenberg, N., Tonegawa, S. and Baltimore, D. (1984). Ordered rearrangement of immunoglobulin heavy chain V segment. *EMBO J.*, **3**, 1209–19

37. Andrade, L., Martinez, C. A. and Coutinho, A. (1988). Mother-derived selection of immune repertoires: non-genetic transmission of developmental choices. In Chaouat, G. (ed.) *The Immunology of the Fetus*, pp. 188–91. (Boca Raton:CRC Press)

38. Martinez, C. A., Marcos, M. A. M., Pereira, P., Marquez, C. and Toribio, P. A. (1986). Turning (Ir-gene) low-responder mice into high responders by antibody manipulation of the developing immune system. *Proc. Natl. Acad. Sci. USA*, **84**, 3812–16

39. Elliot, M. and Kearney, J. F. (1992). Idiotypic regulation of development of the B-cell repertoire. *Ann. N.Y. Acad. Sci.*, **651**, 336–45

40. Martinez-A, C., Pereira, P., Toribio, M. L., Marcos, M. A. R., Bandeira, A., De la Hera, A., Marquez, C., Cazenave, P.-A. and Coutinho, A. (1988). The participation of B cells and antibodies in the selection and maintenance of T cell repertoires. *Immunol. Rev.*, **101**, 191–215

41. Pereira, P., Bandeira, A., Coutinho, A., Marcos, M. A., Toribio, M. and Martinez-A, C. (1989). V-region connectivity in T cell repertoires. *Ann. Rev. Immunol.*, **7**, 209–49

42. Coutinho, A., Forni, L., Holmberg, D., Ivars, F. and Vaz, N. (1984). From an antigen-centered, clonal perspective of immune responses to an organism-centered, network perspective of autonomous activity in a self-referential immune system. *Immunol. Rev.*, **79**, 151–68

43. Vaz, N. M., Martinez, C. A. and Coutinho, A. (1984). The uniqueness and boundaries of the idiotypic self. In Kohler, H., Cazenave, J.-P. and Urbain, J. (eds.) *Idiotypy in Biology and Medicine*. (New York:Academic Press)

44. Dietrich, G., Kaveri, S. V. and Kazatchkine, M. D. (1992). A V-region connected autoreactive subfraction of normal human immunoglobulins G. *Eur. J. Immunol.*, **22**, 1701–6

45. Adib, M., Ragimbeau, J., Avrameas, S. and Ternynck, T. (1990). IgG autoantibody activity in normal mouse serum is controlled by IgM. *J. Immunol.*, **145**, 3807–13

46. Hurez, V., Kaveri, S. V. and Kazatchkine, M. D. (1993). Expression and control of IgG autoreactivity in normal human serum. *Eur. J. Immunol.*, in press

47. McGuire, W. A., Yang, H. H., Bruno, E., Brandt, J., Briddell, R., Coates, T. D. and Hoffman, R. (1987). Treatment of antibody-mediated pure red-cell aplasia with high-dose intravenous γ-globulin. *N. Engl. J. Med.*, **317**, 1004–8

48. Rossi, F. and Kazatchkine, M. D. (1989). Anti-idiotypes against autoantibodies in pooled normal human polyspecific Ig. *J. Immunol.*, **143**, 4104-9

49. van-Doorn, P. A., Rossi, F., Brand, A., Lint, M. V., Vermeulen, M. and Kazatchkine, M. (1990). On the mechanism of high-dose intravenous immunoglobulin treatment of patients with chronic inflammatory demyelinating polyneuropathy with high-dose intravenous immuno-globulins. *J. Neuroimmunol.*, **29**, 57-64

50. Dietrich, G. and Kazatchkine, M. D. (1990). Normal immunoglobulin G (IgG) for therapeutic use (intravenous Ig) contain anti-idiotypic specifi-cities against an immunodominant, disease-associated, cross-reactive idiotype of human anti-thyroglobulin autoantibodies. *J. Clin. Invest.*, **85**, 620-4

51. Marchalonis, J. J., Kaymaz, H., Dedeoglu, F., Schlutter, S. F., Yocum, D. E. and Edmundson, A. B. (1992). Human autoantibodies reactive with synthetic autoantigens from T-cell receptor β chain. *Proc. Natl. Acad. Sci. USA*, **89**, 3325-9

52. Kaveri, S. V., Kang, C. Y. and Kohler, H. (1990). Natural mouse and human antibodies bind to a peptide derived from a germline-variable heavy chain: evidence for evolutionary conserved self-binding locus. *J. Immunol.*, **145**, 4207-13

53. Vassilev, T., Kaveri, S. V., Gelin, C. and Kazatchkine, M. D. (1992). Anti-CD5 antibodies in pooled normal immunoglobulins for ther-apeutic use (intravenous immunoglobulins, IVIG). *Clin. Exp. Immunol.*, in press

54. Zouali, M. and Eyquem, A. (1983). Expression of anti-idiotypic clones against auto-anti-DNA antibodies in normal individuals. *Cell. Immunol.*, **76**, 137-47

55. Dwyer, D. S., Bradley, R. J., Urquhart, C. K. and Kearney, J. F. (1983). Naturally occurring anti-idiotypic antibodies in myasthenia gravis patients. *Nature (London)*, **301**, 611-14

56. Freitas, A. A., Viale, A. C., Sundblad, A., Heusser, C. and Coutinho, A. (1991). Normal serum immunoglobulins participate in the selec-tion of peripheral B-cell repertoires. *Proc. Natl. Acad. Sci. USA*, **88**, 5640-4

57. Sundblad, A., Huetz, F., Portnoï, D. and Coutinho, A. (1991). Stimulation of B and T Cells by *in vivo* high-dose immunoglobulin administration in normal mice. *J. Autoimmun.*, **4**, 325-39

58. Sundblad, A., Marcos, M., Huetz, F., Freitas, A., Heusser, C., Portnoï, D. and Coutinho, A. (1991). Normal serum immunoglobulins influence the numbers of bone marrow pre-B and B cells. *Eur. J. Immunol.*, **21**, 1155-61

59. Dietrich, G., Varela, F., Hurez, V., Bouanani, M. and Kazatchkine, M. D. (1992). Manipulating immune networks with normal immunoglobulin G. *Proc. Natl. Acad. Sci. USA*, in press

60. Varela, F., Anderson, A., Dietrich, G., Sundblad, A., Holmberg, D., Kazatchkine, M. D. and Coutinho, A. (1991). The population dynamics of antibodies in normal and autoimmune individuals. *Proc. Natl. Acad. Sci. USA*, **88,** 5917–21

10

Immunoglobulins in severe viral pediatric disease

F. J. Leal

Despite all the progress made in the development of antiviral agents, clinicians are frequently faced with severe viral disease conditions for which there is no effective agent available. However, it has been suggested that serious viral disease is a depletion-associated antibody immunodeficiency. Some such life-threatening diseases, therefore, may respond to intravenous immunoglobulin supplementation (IVIG)[1]. Although the nature of this therapeutic approach only admits isolated reports, we have carried out a review of the subject, including our own experience, in the conviction that the information thus gathered may be found helpful in many similar clinical situations. The results may be summarized as follows.

VARICELLA

The prevention of varicella by IVIG has been considered in immuno-compromised children. This use of IVIG may also be effective in the correction of postviral thrombocytopenia. Neonatal varicella, which leads to visceral involvement and death, may be prevented or its course may be altered by hyperimmune γ-globulin. It has been suggested that IVIG is helpful in very small neonates with low muscle mass[2].

RUBEOLA

In spite of the significant risk of embryopathy, it is hard to prevent it in those countries whose legislation does not permit therapeutic abortion, and even where this procedure is legal, many women themselves reject it on religious grounds. Standard intramuscular γ-globulin has not proved to be effective. Specific hyperimmune γ-globulin is not available. The efficacy of IVIG remains to be established[3].

POLIO

Although passive immunization may provide protection for 6–8 weeks, active immunization is the best prophylactic method. Since hypogammaglobulinemic individuals present with a life-threatening clinical picture[4], antibodies are supposed to be useful. We observed a hypogammaglobulinemic patient vaccinated with live virus, who developed a severe condition requiring assisted ventilation. After being given IVIG, the patient improved dramatically; no sequelae were noted, except for a slight pretibial paresis.

RESPIRATORY VIRUSES

Animal studies have shown that IVIG may be useful for prevention and treatment of respiratory syncytial virus (RSV) infections. Children with RSV pneumonia show significant reductions in virus counts and improved oxygenation[5]. Our review includes non-controlled studies of adenovirus pneumonia in immunocompromised individuals who showed a favorable clinical course[2].

ENTEROVIRUSES

Although the role of antibodies in these cases is unclear, IVIG has been effective in controlling the infection in agammaglobulinemic patients with meningoencephalitis due to echovirus 11, whether alone or in conjunction with myositis-fascitis[6,7]. A similar experience has been reported with coxsackievirus infection.

CYTOMEGALOVIRUS

Cytomegalovirus (CMV) infection is common in neonates and it carries significant morbidity and mortality. It has been noted that IVIG is useful in recipients of bone marrow transplants[8]. It has been also effective in patients with thrombocytopenia following CMV infection.

OTHER VIRAL CONDITIONS

The efficacy of IVIG in pediatric acquired immune deficiency syndrome (AIDS) is well known. Equally well established is its beneficial action in another severe entity possibly due to a viral pathogen, namely the Kawasaki syndrome[9]. A non-controlled study has reported the clinical efficacy of IVIG in eight out of 12 patients with chronic infection due to Epstein–Barr virus[10]. Another report describes a case of thrombocytopenia which improved significantly after IVIG was added to acyclovir[11]. The agent has also been found useful in recurring genital herpes. Lastly, it may be beneficial in infectious conditions due to parvovirus B19, because the batches show adequate titers[12].

IVIG may be a valuable therapeutic agent in a number of severe viral pediatric diseases. However, careful clinical observation is needed to establish its real efficacy.

REFERENCES

1. Stiehm, E. R. (1991). Use of immunoglobulin therapy in secondary antibody deficiencies. In Imbach, P. (ed.) *Immunotherapy with Intravenous Immunoglobulins*, pp. 115–26. (London:Academic Press)
2. Fisher, G. W. (1988). *Gammaglobulin Therapy in the Treatment and Prevention of Viral Illnesses*, pp. 55–72. (American Association of Blood Banks)
3. Plotkin, S. A. (1973). In Plotkin, S. A. and Mortimer, E. A. (eds.) *Rubella Vaccine*, p. 241. (Philadelphia:Saunders)
4. Wyatt, H. V. (1973). Poliomyelitis in hypogammaglobulinemics. *J. Infect. Dis.*, **128**, 802–6
5. Hemming, V. G. and Prince, G. A. (1991). Passive immunization for the protection of infants and young children from respiratory infection by respiratory synctial virus. In Imbach, P. (ed.) *Immunotherapy with Intravenous Immunoglobulins*, pp. 103–12. (London:Academic Press)

6. Webster, A. D. B., Hayward, A. B. *et al.* (1988). Echovirus encephalitis and myostitis in primary immunoglobulin deficiency. *Arch. Dis. Child.*, **53**, 33–7
7. Erlendsson, K., Swartz, T. and Dwyer, J. M. (1985). Successful reversal of echovirus in X-linked hypogammaglobulinemia by intraventricular administration of immunoglobulin. *N. Engl. J. Med.*, **312**, 351–3
8. Elfenbein, G., Krisher, J., Graham-Pole, J. *et al.* (1991). Intravenous immunoglobulin for cytomegalovirus pneumonia. In Imbach P. (ed.) *Immunotherapy with Intravenous Immunoglobulin*, pp. 219–28. (London: Academic Press)
9. Furusto, K., Sato, K. *et al.* (1983). High-dose intravenous gammaglobulin for Kawasaki disease. *Lancet*, **2**, 1359
10. Tobi, M. and Straus, S. E. (1985). Chronic Epstein–Barr virus disease: a workshop held by the National Institute of Allergy and Infectious Diseases. *Ann. Intern. Med.*, **103**, 951–2
11. Hugo, M., Linde, A. and Abom, P. (1989). Epstein–Barr virus induced thrombocytopenia treated with intravenous acyclovir and immuno-globulin. *Scand. J. Infect. Dis.*, **21**, 103–5
12. Schwarz, T. F., Raggendorf, M., Hottentrager, B. *et al.* (1990). Immunoglobulin in the prophylaxis of parvovirus B19 infection. *J. Immunol. Dis.*, **162**, 1214

11

Immune thrombocytopenia and mononuclear phagocyte function

A. C. Newland and M. G. Macey

INTRODUCTION

Platelet destruction in immune thrombocytopenia (ITP) results from the binding of antibody to a platelet-associated antigen, with or without complement activation, followed by phagocytosis. This latter is triggered by the Fc portion of the IgG molecule, or by complement activation with C3b fixation to the cell surface[1]. The Fc mechanism is important in the pathogenesis of ITP. Platelet destruction takes place primarily in the mononuclear phagocyte system (MPS)[2,3]. For optimal platelet destruction there must be sufficient quantities of antigen, antibody and phagocytic cells with sufficient time for binding to occur for subsequent platelet phagocytosis. This occurs primarily in three organs, the spleen, the liver and the bone marrow.

Of these, the spleen is optimally suited, as one-third of the platelet mass is present in the spleen at all times. Splenic blood flow allows antibody-coated platelets to circulate slowly through the dense reticular network with its large phagocytic component. In addition, it has been shown that an antiplatelet antibody is secreted in the spleen, so that intrasplenic platelets are subject to higher antibody concentrations than those in the plasma[4]. The liver, by contrast, contains no significant platelet pool, produces no significant antiplatelet antibody, and has a more rapid circulation. It is therefore less involved in pathological platelet destruction than the spleen[5,6]. The role of the bone marrow is less clear. Bone marrow has a large megakaryocyte population and, although platelet turnover is generally regarded as normal or increased in ITP[6-9] this may not always be the case. There is some evidence suggesting that there may be damage to megakaryocytes by antiplatelet antibody[10]. *In vitro* studies have also shown evidence for local platelet uptake by marrow phagocytic cells[11]. It has also been shown that, following splenectomy, the bone marrow is the most likely source of antiplatelet antibody[12].

Shulman and co-workers[2], in 1965, demonstrated that patients with hereditary spherocytosis were relatively resistant to the development of thrombocytopenia caused by infusion of ITP plasma. He speculated that excessive uptake of red blood cells by the MPS interfered with platelet sequestration. He also demonstrated that infusion of autologous red cell stroma in normal subjects inhibited the same phenomenon. These observations highlighted the MPS as the final common pathway for platelet phagocytosis and destruction.

Following the initial therapeutic impact of intravenous immunoglobulin (IVIG) in ITP, attention focused on Fc-receptor (FcR) blockade as the mechanism of platelet response. This effect had originally been demonstrated for glucocorticoids[13] showing a relationship between neutrophil phagocytosis, the platelet count and the prednisolone dose. A subsequent study of IVIG suggested that its effects, as quantified by antibody-coated autologous red cell clearance, were more profound than were those of steroids[14].

Earlier studies of the effects of IgG[15,16] and immune complexes[17] on Fc-mediated phagocytosis had already suggested this as a possible mechanism of action. Aggregated IgG and immune complexes were shown to inhibit Fc-mediated phagocytosis of IgG-coated red cells[18].

Our study looked at various aspects of MPS function. The MPS participates in several well-defined functions, including inflammation, antimicrobial activity, the immune response and the clearance of foreign substances and debris. The capacity for phagocytosis is one of the primary characteristics, however, and it is important in the clearance of foreign or abnormal substances from the circulation, or from a local tissue site. This may be achieved by two main mechanisms, non-specific ingestion of substances such as latex particles, zymosan, yeast capsules or certain bacteria, and specific ingestion, which occurs via surface receptors, including the receptor for the Fc region of the immunoglobulin and the receptor for complement component C3b[19]. The suggestion is that the use of IVIG blocks such specific ingestion, and is the pathway for the early response.

However, it is possible that non–specific ingestion may be stimulated by the infusion of high doses of immunoglobulin. These contain small concentrations of aggregates and may form immune complexes once in the circulation; these are known to be responsible for monocyte activation[20,21], possibly by cytokine release. Such activation has been indicated by an increase in lactate dehydrogenase levels[22] and by the increased red cell destruction seen in some patients[23]. Such differential effects may explain the unpredictable clinical response following IVIG.

Studies were undertaken using both antibody-coated red cells and heat-damaged red cells *in vivo* to monitor both Fc-specific mediated particle clearance and non-specific function. These studies were supported by *in vitro* observations on the ability of patients' neutrophils to phagocytose opsonized autologous platelets during IVIG treatment.

PLATELET PHAGOCYTOSIS

Platelet phagocytosis by patients' neutrophils was measured using opsonized autologous platelets in nine patients. There was a marked reduction in platelet phagocytosis as measured by formazan production

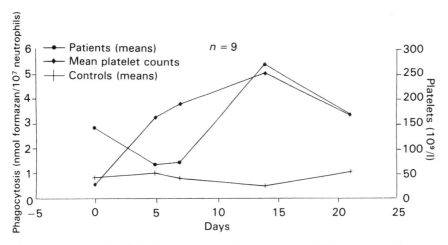

Figure 1 Mean value of platelet phagocytosis by patient neutrophils (intravenous immunoglobulin, days 1-5)

in all patients at days 4–5, compared with the preinfusion value, and in half of these, this reduction was still evident at further studies 1 week after the end of the infusion period. In the majority, the phagocytic ability had returned to pretreatment values 2 or 3 weeks after the end of the infusion, and in some there was quite a marked overshoot in measured phagocytic ability (Figure 1). Each study was done in parallel with a control sample using neutrophils from a normal subject. The normal range was calculated using samples from 20 controls, and the result of 0.68 ± 0.17 (mean $\pm$ SE) is close to the prevalue mean for controls of 0.7. In this study three patients were receiving no treatment, the rest were all receiving prednisolone, and the results do not differ between these two groups. The platelet count rose in parallel with the fall in platelet phagocytic ability of the neutrophils, reaching a peak at 7 days postinfusion, and fell with the recovery of phagocytic function in weeks 2 and 3. The fall in platelet count lagged behind the recovering function by several days. The control values did not alter significantly during the study period.

HEAT-DAMAGED AUTOLOGOUS RED CELL CLEARANCE

Clearance of heat-damaged red blood cells (HDRBC) labelled with technetium-99M (^{99M}Tc) was carried out in eight patients before and

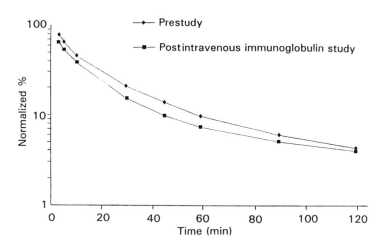

Figure 2   Heat-damaged autologous red blood cell clearance

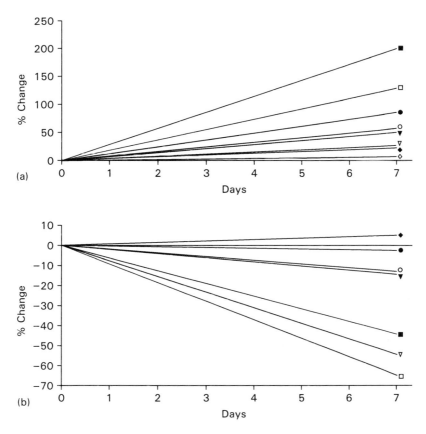

Figure 3 (a) Percentage change in heat-damaged red blood cell clearance C20-splenic function. (b) Percentage change in heat-damaged red blood cell clearance %60 – irreversible cell removal. Each symbol represents an individual patient

after a 5-day infusion of IVIG. All had their spleens present at the time of the study. The results were plotted as a clearance curve on semi-logarithmic paper, and a typical example is shown in Figure 2. In the great majority of patients the curves obtained were of the form predicted in the original studies of Peters and colleagues[24], although in at least four of the studies the clearance time was so slow that the calculation of the time taken for the value at 3 min to fall by 50% ($T_{0.5}$) was not possible. This is a measure of liver clearance. In six of the eight, the curves showed enhanced post-IVIG clearance of HDRBC.

121

The percentage fall in the clearance curve between 8 and 28 min (C20) was measured. Peters and co-workers[25] had shown that this correlates with splenic determinants of HDRBC clearance, particularly phagocytosis and splenic blood flow. Unlike the $T_{0.5}$, it is less affected by liver clearance. The mean value in normal subjects at 30 min after the 8-min value is $41 \pm 12\%$ in normal subjects. This is equivalent to the C20 in our study. All values of C20 were increased postinfusion, reflecting enhanced splenic function. Thus, the preinfusion mean C20 was 21.8%, increasing to 32.7% postinfusion for the group as a whole (Figure 3a). The improvement in splenic function as measured by C20 was paralleled by a reduction in the percentage of radiolabelled HDRBC left at 60 min (%60), which is a measure of irreversible cell removal (Figure 3b). All but one of the patients showed a reduction in %60, the mean falling from 59.5 to 46.4. There was no correlation between the percentage change of C20 compared to a percentage change of %60, but in general as the measure of splenic blood flow and phagocytosis increased the irreversible clearance of HDRBC was also enhanced.

ANTI-D-COATED TECHNETIUM-LABELLED RED BLOOD CELL CLEARANCE STUDIES

Clearance studies were performed in eight Rh-D-positive patients using autologous red cells coated with anti-D and labelled with ^{99M}Tc.

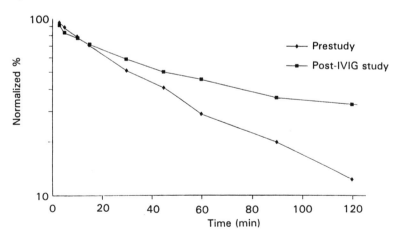

Figure 4 Anti-D-labelled autologous red blood cell clearance

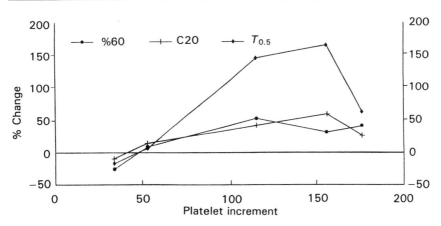

Figure 5 Percentage change in anti-D-labelled red blood cell survival compared to response

Pre- and poststudies were performed in all patients, and in one with chronic ITP a further study was performed at 3 weeks. A typical study is shown in Figure 4. As with the previous study, the measurements of $T_{0.5}$, C20 and %60 were determined and are presented in Figure 5. $T_{0.5}$ increased in seven of the eight patients, from a mean of 78.5 min to 137.1 min, a prolongation of 74.6%. The patient in whom the $T_{0.5}$ reduced also showed only a minor response in platelet increment.

Splenic function, as measured by C20, showed a reduction in all but one of the patients studied following IVIG. The one exception also showed enhancement of general MPS function as measured by $T_{0.5}$, and cleared a higher percentage of anti-D-labelled cells as measured by the %60. All other patients showed delayed clearance of radiolabelled cells as measured by the %60 which is a measure of irreversible cell damage. In general, reduced MPS function as measured by the $T_{0.5}$ correlated with reduced splenic function as measured by the C20, and was paralleled with a reduction in clearance of labelled cells. There was an association between these changes and the subsequent platelet increment following IVIG (Figure 5).

NEUTROPHIL COUNT

The neutrophil count was recorded in a cohort of 40 patients with ITP treated with IVIG. Counts were taken immediately prior to the first infusion of IVIG and on either the last day or the day after the final

123

Table 1 Relationship between neutrophil decrease and platelet increase in immune thrombocytopenia treated with intravenous immunoglobulin

Platelet response ($\times 10^9$/l)	Mean platelet rise	Mean neutrophil fall (range)
Good responders (n = 13)		
>150	222	−2.99
		(−0.64 to −8.47)
Moderate responders (n = 9)		
>100	126	−1.50
		(−0.81 to −2.32)
Intermediate (n = 15)		
30–100	64	−1.11
		(+0.90 to −2.90)
Poor responders (n = 3)		
<30	13	+0.89
		(+1.58 to −0.46)

infusion. Thirty-six showed a reduction in the neutrophil count over the period of infusion. The decrease was significant ($p < 0.001$) from the count before treatment, mean 6.25×10^9/l to that on days 4/5 of the treatment (mean 4.57×10^9/l). The data are not shown, but the neutropenic period was brief, the counts returning to normal by 7 days after treatment. The reduction was associated with an increase in platelet count (mean 125×10^9/l), increasing from 33×10^9/l preinfusion to 158×10^9/l immediately afterwards. There was a correlation ($p < 0.01$) between the decrease in neutrophil count and the increase in the platelet count, and when the platelet increment was analyzed according to degree (>150, >100, 30–100, <30) there was a close correlation between the response and degree of neutropenia observed (Table 1).

DISCUSSION

The results of these studies on MPS activity suggest that IVIG has a marked influence on the body's phagocytic ability. Enhanced platelet phagocytosis-measured preinfusion confirms the increased phagocytic potential that would be expected in patients with uncontrolled peripheral platelet destruction. However, following IVIG the phagocytosis of autologous platelets by the patient's neutrophils was impaired. With other studies (not reported here) showing reduced phagocytosis of bacteria, the suggestion is that IVIG has a direct inhibitory effect on neutrophil function.

Abe and Matsuda[26] also studied the effect of IVIG on the uptake of *Escherichia coli* by neutrophils using a chemiluminescent assay. They showed that the *in vitro* uptake of opsonized *E. coli* by the neutrophils from normal individuals and patients with hemophilia was reduced during IVIG infusion. Similar results were also obtained in an *in vivo* study by the same group, when they monitored the phagocytic ability of patient neutrophils pre- and post-IVIG infusion. In all cases studied, the phagocytic ability was reduced after the infusion, confirming the findings of the current study.

The results of MPS function as measured by the clearance rate of red blood cells varied according to the technique used. The rate of clearance from the blood of radiolabelled autologous HDRBC is an acknowledged test of splenic function[27], and has been used to monitor diseases which, it has been claimed, cause saturation and impairment of macrophage function[28]. HDRBC are trapped by the microvasculature of the spleen, delaying transit time. The cells will then either ultimately re-enter the circulation, or be irreversibly trapped and taken up by splenic macrophages. The rate of decay of radioactivity in the blood is a measure of this irreversible uptake, and can be used to quantify splenic function. In six of the eight patients studied before IVIG infusion, the rate of clearance of the HDRBC was greatly prolonged, above the normal range, suggesting macrophage saturation. However, following IVIG the clearance time became marginally shorter in six of the eight, suggesting that high doses of IVIG may enhance non-specific macrophage function. Other workers[29] have shown that following IVIG there is a marked increase in intracellular IgG in the mononuclear cells. The possibility is, therefore, that the large increase in serum IgG is accompanied by the transient increase in membrane-bound IgG, which is then rapidly internalized[30], and that the process of internalization of IgG aggregates enhances non-specific cellular phagocytosis.

The results using anti-D-coated radiolabelled red cells are markedly different. The majority of patients show a significant delay in antibody-coated red cell clearance following IVIG. Functional data are available that show that the differential clearance of antibody-coated and HDRBC is different; the former is suppressible by steroids, whereas the latter is not[31]. Anti-D-coated red blood cells are a model system for measuring MPS Fc function, and the prolongation of clearance in these and other studies suggests that the Fc receptors on the MPS are functionally blocked by the infusion of IVIG, as has already been suggested. Monomeric IgG can inhibit Fc receptor–ligand interactions[32,33]. Following IVIG, the *in vivo* serum concentration of monomeric IgG may increase threefold, and might enhance the competition between monomeric IgG with immunologically sensitized platelets or red cells for Fc receptors, thus delaying their removal. IVIG is also known to contain more aggregates[34], and these are known to block Fc function in the animal model[35,36]. Thus, following IVIG there is a transient dysfunction of Fc-mediated hepatic and splenic MPS clearance, accompanied by a variable increase in the platelet count.

The *in vitro* and *in vivo* studies suggest that the basis for these effects is altered phagocyte–target interaction, due to a decreased Fc-mediated phagocytic capacity. The marked increase in intracellular IgG measured[29] is associated with the decrease in Fc rosettes, and is consistent with the hypothesis of phagocytosis and internalization of Fc receptors, with the concomitant reduction in Fc function. It therefore appears that IVIG selectively blocks Fc-mediated MPS function, while at the same time enhancing non-specific phagocytic clearance. The latter is not, however, associated with any change in the platelet count in these patients, but the variable effect observed might explain the different increments seen between patients and at different times following infusion in the same patient.

During treatment the majority of patients studied exhibited a mild neutropenia. The reduction in neutrophil count may be due to activation of the neutrophil, with subsequent removal from circulation. Neutrophils have both high-affinity (FcR2) and low-affinity (FcR3) Fc receptors[37]. Neither receptor binds monomeric IgG, but does bind dimers, aggregates and immune complexes, and IVIG has been shown to contain small amounts of aggregates and up to 40% dimers[38]. The flow cytometric analysis of the neutrophil surface during IVIG infusion shows increased surface-bound IgG compared to pretreatment[39,40]. *In vitro* studies of the binding of IVIG to neutrophils in relation to the

126

expression of the FcR3 receptor have been performed, and these show that the expression of FcR3 varies in a reciprocal manner to the amount of neutrophil surface-bound IgG. This suggests that IgG aggregates in the IVIG were binding to the FcR3. Ultracentrifugation of IVIG to remove IgG aggregates before testing reduces the amount of IgG binding *in vitro*[39].

These findings support the hypothesis that the clinical response to IVIG is in part due to the binding of IgG to the Fc receptors, resulting in altered Fc-mediated phagocytosis in both the circulating and tissue-bound mononuclear phagocyte systems.

REFERENCES

1. Stossel, T. P. (1974). Phagocytosis. *N. Engl. J. Med.*, **290**, 717–23; 774–80; 833–9
2. Shulman, N. R., Weinrach, R. S., Libre, E. P. and Andrews, H. L. (1965). The role of the reticuloendothelial system in the pathogenesis of idiopathic thrombocytopenic purpura. *Trans. Assoc. Am. Physicians*, **78**, 374–89
3. McMillan, R., Longmire, R. L., Tavassoli, M., Armstrong, S. and Yelenosky, R. (1974). *In vitro* platelet phagocytosis by splenic leukocytes in idiopathic thrombocytopenic purpura. *N. Engl. J. Med.*, **290**, 249–51
4. McMillan, R., Martin, M., Bakich, M. J. and Morrison, J. (1979). A new assay for the evaluation of antiplatelet antibody in idiopathic thrombocytopenic purpura. *Immunopharmacology*, **1**, 83–7
5. Aster, R. H. (1966). Pooling of platelets in the spleen: role of the pathogenesis of 'hypersplenic' thrombocytopenia. *J. Clin. Invest.*, **45**, 645–57
6. Aster, R. H. and Keene, W. R. (1969). Sites of platelet destruction in idiopathic thrombocytopenic purpura. *Br. J. Haematol.*, **16**, 61–73
7. Harker, L. A. (1970). Thrombokinetics in idiopathic thrombocytopenic purpura. *Br. J. Haematol.*, **19**, 95–104
8. Branehog, I., Kutti, J. and Weinfeld, A. (1974). Platelet survival and platelet production in idiopathic thrombocytopenic purpura. *Br. J. Haematol.*, **27**, 127–43
9. Najean, Y., Ardaillou, N., Caen, J., Larrien, M. J. and Bernard, J. (1963). Survival of radiochromium C-labelled platelets in thrombocytopenia. *Blood*, **22**, 718–32
10. Heyns, A. du P., Badenhorst, P. N., Lotter, M. G., Pieters, H., Wessels, P. and Kotze, H. F. (1986). Platelet turnover and kinetics in immune thrombocytopenic purpura: results with autologous ^{111}In-labeled platelets and homologous ^{51}Cr-labeled platelets differ. *Blood*, **67**, 86–92

11. Izak, G. and Nelken, D. (1957). Studies in thrombopoiesis *in vitro* from the bone marrow of patients with idiopathic thrombocytopenic purpura. *Blood*, **12**, 520–8

12. McMillan, R., Yelenosky, R. J. and Longmire, R. L. (1976). Antiplatelet antibody production by the spleen and bone marrow in immune thrombocytopenic purpura. In Battisto, J. R. and Streilein, J. W. (eds.) *Immuno Aspects of the Spleen*, pp. 227–37. (Amsterdam:North Holland)

13. Robson, H. N. and Duthie, J. J. R. (1950). Capillary resistance and adrenocortical activity. *Br. Med. J.*, **2**, 971

14. Fehr, J., Hofmann, V. and Kappeler, U. (1982). Transient reversal of thrombocytopenia in idiopathic thrombocytopenic purpura by high-dose intravenous γ-globulin. *N. Engl. J. Med.*, **306**, 1254–8

15. Huber, H. and Fudenberg, H. H. (1968). Receptor sites of human monocytes for IgG. *Int. Arch. Allergy*, **34**, 18–31

16. Williams, A. J., Hastings, M. G. G., Easman, C. S. F. and Cole, P. J. (1980). Factors affecting the *in vitro* assessment of opsonisation: a study of the kinetics of opsonisation using the technique of phagocytic chemiluminescence. *Immunology*, **41**, 903–11

17. Griffin, F. M. (1980). Effects of soluble immune complexes on Fc receptor mediated phagocytosis by macrophages. *J. Exp. Med.*, **152**, 905–19

18. Fleer, A., Meullen Van der, F. W., Linthout Els, Von dem Borne, A. E. G. Kr. and Engelfriet, A. (1978). Destruction of IgG sensitized erythrocytes by human blood monocytes: modulation of inhibition by IgG. *Br. J. Haematol.*, **39**, 425–36

19. Kimberly, R. P. and Ralph, P. (1983). Endocytosis by the mononuclear phagocyte system and autoimmune disease. *Am. J. Med.*, **74**, 481–93

20. Karnovsky, M. and Lazdins, J. K. (1978). Biochemical criteria for activated monocytes. *J. Immunol.*, **121**, 808

21. Pestel, J., Joseph, M., Dessaint, J. and Capron, A. (1981). Macrophage triggering by aggregated immunoglobulins (i) Delayed effect of IgG aggregates on immune complexes. *J. Immunol.*, **126**, 1887

22. Kavai, M., Zsindely, D., Sonkoly, I., Major, M., Demjan, I. and Szegedi, G. (1983). Signals of monocyte activation in patients with SLE. *Clin. Exp. Immunol.*, **51**, 255–60

23. Copelan, E. A., Strohm, P. L., Kennedy, M. S. and Tutschka, P. J. (1986). Haemolysis following intravenous immunoglobulin therapy. *Transfusion*, **26**, 410–12

24. Peters, A. M., Ryan, P. F. J., Klonizakis, I., Elkon, K. B., Lewis, S. M. and Hughes, G. R. V. (1981). Analysis of heat-damaged erythrocyte clearance curves. *Br. J. Haematol.*, **49**, 581–6

25. Peters, A. M., Ryan, P. F. J., Klonizakis, I., Elkon, K. B., Lewis, S. M. and Hughes, G. R. V. (1981). Measurement of splenic function in humans using heat damaged autologous red blood cells. *Scand. J. Haematol.*, **27**, 374–80

26. Abe, T. and Matsuda, J. (1986). Effects of immunoglobulin on cellular and humoral immunity of haemophiliacs with reversed T4/T8 ratio of lymphocytes. In Morrel, A. and Nydegger, U. E. (eds.) *Clinical Uses of Intravenous Immunoglobulins*, pp. 385–98. (London:Academic Press)

27. Petitt, J. E. (1977). Splenic function. *Clinics in Haematology*, **6**, 639–56

28. Lockwood, C. M., Worlledge, S., Nicholas, A., Cotton, C. and Peters, D. K. (1979). Reversal of impaired splenic function in patients with nephritis or vasculitis (or both) by plasma exchange. *N. Engl. J. Med.*, **300**, 524–30

29. Kimberly, R. P., Salmon, J. E., Bussel, J. B., Crow, M. K. and Hilgartner, M. W. (1984). Modulation of mononuclear phagocyte function by intravenous γ-globulin. *J. Immunol.*, **132**, 745–50

30. Segal, D. M., Dower, S. K. and Titus, J. A. (1983). The FcR mediated endocytosis of model immune complexes by cells from the P388D1 mouse macrophage cell line. I. Internalisation of small, non-aggregating oligomers of IgG. *J. Immunol.*, **130**, 130–7

31. Klausner, M. A., Hirsch, L. J., Leblond, P. F., Chamberlain, J. K., Klemperer, M. R. and Segel, G. B. (1975). Contrasting splenic mechanisms in the blood clearance of red blood cells and colloidal particles. *Blood*, **46**, 965–76

32. Kurlander, R. J. (1980). Reversible and irreversible loss of Fc receptor function of human monocytes as a consequence of interaction with immunoglobulin G. *J. Clin. Invest.*, **66**, 773–81

33. Segal, D. M., Titus, J. A. and Dower, S. K. (1983). The FcR mediated endocytosis of model immune complexes by cells from the P388D1 mouse macrophage cell line. II. The role of ligand-induced self-aggregation in promoting internalisation. *J. Immunol.*, **130**, 138

34. Romer, J., Morgenthaler, J. J., Scherz, R. and Skvarilk, F. (1982). Characterisation of various immunoglobulin preparations for intravenous application. I. Protein composition and antibody content. *Vox Sang.*, **42**, 62–78

35. Haakenstad, A. O. and Mannik, M. (1974). Saturation of the reticuloendothelial system with soluble immune complexes. *J. Immunol.*, **112**, 1939–48

36. Lawrence, S., Lockwood, C. M. and Peters, D. K. (1981). Studies on NEM-treated erythrocyte clearance in the rabbit with special reference to the effects of circulating immune complexes. *Clin. Exp. Immunol.*, **44**, 433

37. Anderson, C. C. and Looney, A. J. (1986). Human leukocyte IgG Fc receptors. *Immunol. Today*, **7**, 246–66

38. Tankersley, D. L., Preston, M. S. and Finlanson, J. S. (1988). Immuno-globulin G dimer: an idiotype–antiidiotype complex. *Mol. Immunol.*, **25**, 41–8
39. Veys, P. A., Gutteridge, C. N., Macey, M. G., Ord, J. and Newland, A. C. (1989). The detection of granulocyte antibodies using flow cytometric analysis of leukocyte immunofluorescence. *Vox Sang.*, **56**, 42–7
40. Minchinton, R. M. and McGrath, K. (1987). Binding and antibody block-ing effects of intravenous IgG preparations on peripheral blood cells. *Clin. Lab. Haematol.*, **9**, 49–58

12

Management of immune thrombocytopenic purpura and other immunological cytopenias with human intravenous immunoglobulins

P. A. Imbach

INTRODUCTION

In idiopathic (immune) thrombocytopenic purpura (ITP) two controversial effects of immunoglobulins have to be considered: first, the thrombocytopenic effect if antibodies (immunoglobulins) from patients with chronic ITP are administered to volunteers with normal platelet counts[1], and secondly, the increasing effect on platelet count when pooled immunoglobulins from healthy blood donors are given to patients with ITP[2]. Immune cytopenias present either as acute postinfectious disorders or as chronic autoimmune disease. What are the pathogenetic events? What are the target antigens? How can these disorders be influenced by intravenous immunoglobulin (IVIG)? These questions will be discussed in this chapter.

VIRUS-INDUCED AUTOIMMUNE PHENOMENONA ON BLOOD CELLS

Immune cytopenias are disorders characterized by increased destruction of circulating erythrocytes, neutrophils and/or platelets. Antibodies provoke the early destruction of blood cells. The appearance of

Table 1 Virus-induced autoimmunity

	Erythrocytes	Leukocytes	Thrombocytes	Bone marrow cells
Measles*			+	+
Mumps			(+)	
Rubella*			+	+
Hepatitis A			(+)	+
HIV		+	+	
EBV	+		+	+
CMV	+	+	+	+
B19	+	+	+	+

*, Also after vaccination; (+), Mild autoimmunity; HIV, human immuno-deficiency virus; EBV, Epstein–Barr virus; CMV, cytomegalovirus

antibodies against blood cells is often associated with viral infections. Some of these viral infections, which may induce immunocytopenia, are listed in Table 1. After infections such as measles, mumps and rubella, or after antiviral vaccination, antibodies against platelets, neutrophils and red cells with no antigen specificity have been noted to appear[3,4] and increased numbers of circulating activated T cells have been observed[5]. In children with human immunodeficiency virus (HIV) infection after maternofetal transmission or blood transfusion-related transmission, thrombocytopenia has been estimated to occur in about 40% of cases[6]. Specific antiplatelet antibodies[7,8], as well as circulating[9] or platelet-bound immune complexes[10], have been demonstrated in such conditions. Mega-karyocytes may contain HIV-related ribonucleic acid, which suggests a direct involvement of progenitor cells in the development of thrombo-cytopenia[11]. Neutropenia becomes more severe with progression of the HIV infection[12-14]. The production of antiplatelet and antineutrophil antibodies seems to be due primarily to B-cell polyclonal activation by HIV[15]. Epstein–Barr viruses (EBV) stimulate B lymphocytes to enhanced production of antibodies which cross-react with normal tissue proteins, exhibiting configurations similar to those of the infectious agent[16]. This corresponds to molecular mimicry. Agranulocytosis due to EBV infection has been observed also in conjunction with bone marrow hypoplasia[17]. Cytomegalovirus (CMV) protein is similar to the human leukocyte antigen (HLA)-DR β-chain protein, and shares a common epitope with it[18]. Thrombocytopenia has been observed in both congenital and acquired CMV infection. CMV infection is known to induce multiple autoantibodies[19]. Human CMV can suppress hematopoiesis[20]. Human parvovirus (B19) inhibits hematopoietic colony formation *in vitro*. Thrombocytopenia, neutropenia and erythrocytopenia, as well as pancytopenia due to parvovirus infection have been reported[21-25].

In ITP, the epitope-directed virally induced autoantibodies are often located on the glycoprotein IIb/IIIa complex on the platelets. In sensitive assays using monoclonal autoantibodies it was possible to detect platelet-associated and plasma autoantibodies[26,27]. Platelet-associated autoantibodies against glycoprotein IIb/IIIa were found in 80% of adults with chronic ITP, and plasma autoantibodies in about half of these patients[28]. In children with chronic ITP, platelet-associated autoantibodies against glycoprotein IIb/IIIa complex could be detected in 72% of patients with ongoing chronic ITP, and in 48% of children with a history of chronic ITP[29]. The detection of autoantibodies against blood cells changed the definition of ITP to immune or autoimmune thrombocytopenia (AITP). As in autoimmune hemolytic anemia (AIHA) and in autoimmune neutropenia (AIN), the rapid destruction of platelets is due to autoantibodies which bind via $F(ab')_2$ to the antigenic site, or to immune complexes which bind via Fc receptors on the platelets. These opsonized cells are rapidly removed by cells of the mononuclear phagocytic system, particularly in the spleen.

IMPLICATIONS OF VIRAL INFECTION ON THE IMMUNE SYSTEM AND POSSIBLE MECHANISMS OF ACTION OF IVIG

Viral disease may change the complex immune response of the host on different levels. Antigen-presenting cells may be disturbed; T cells may be influenced by altered cytokine production and release, thus disturbing the further activation of the network of the immune system; B cells may produce increased amounts of antibodies and, as one of the consequences, the feedback mechanism of the immune system may be 'dysregulated' (Figure 1).

When immunoglobulins from healthy blood donors which contain innumerable different antibodies are administered to an individual with

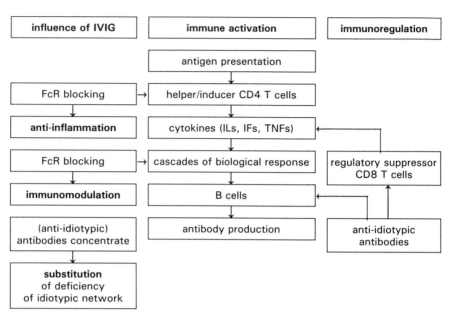

Figure 1 Immune response and possible mechanism of action of intravenous immuno-globulin (IVIG). IL, interleukin; IF, interferon; TNF, tumor necrosis factor; FcR, Fc receptor

an unbalanced immune response, the modes of action of IVIG may be multiple. Each step of the above-mentioned immune response may be influenced, resulting in a more balanced immune response[30].

THERAPEUTIC ASPECTS OF IMMUNE CYTOPENIAS WITH IVIG

Immune thrombocytopenic purpura

This was the first cytopenia to be treated by IVIG. The first observation relates to an 11-year-old boy, who had had life-threatening bleeding episodes despite splenectomy and long-term immunosuppressive treatment. The therapeutic immunosuppression caused a secondary hypo-gammaglobulinemia, for which the boy received IVIG (Sandoglobulin®, Sandoz). Within 24 h after the initial dose of 0.4 g/kg body weight his platelet count increased dramatically. After receiving five doses of IVIG the boy's platelet count rose to over $300 \times 10^9/l$ within 10 days. The same phenomenon was observed in 12 normogammaglobulinemic children with ITP who consecutively received the same dose of IVIG in a pilot study[2]. Thereafter, the platelet-increasing effect of IVIG was studied by controlled multicenter clinical studies, separating children with newly diagnosed ITP from those with chronic ITP[31,32]. The main conclusions from these studies were the following:

(1)   A rapid increase in platelet count was observed within 24–72 h in most patients with acute or chronic ITP;

(2)   In children with chronic ITP, long-term improvement (no more bleeding episodes and platelet counts above $20 \times 10^9/l$) was observed in 62% of patients within an observation time longer than 2 years; and

(3)   The total dosage of 2 g (5×0.4 g) IVIG/kg body weight was too high in two out of three patients.

The reduction to a total initial dose of 2×0.4 g or 1×0.8 g IVIG/kg body weight gave similar results in patients with newly diagnosed acute ITP (with bleeding symptoms and platelet counts below $30 \times 10^9/l$

Table 2 Treatment of idiopathic thrombocytopenia with intravenous immunoglobulin (IVIG)

Initial
Day 1: 0.8 g IVIG/kg body weight
Day 3: – if platelet count is $>30 \times 10^9/l$: no further treatment
          – if platelet count is $<30 \times 10^9/l$: repeat IVIG as on day 1
          – if platelet count is $<10 \times 10^9/l$: bone marrow analysis for exclusion of production disorders of platelets, leukemia etc.

Emergency (severe bleeding, presurgery)
1–2×1.0 g IVIG/kg body weight until platelet counts are at least $>30 \times 10^9/l$ or there is no more bleeding. Eventually combination with high-dose methylprednisolone (8–12 mg/kg body weight intravenously or orally) and/or with platelet transfusion

Chronic ITP (platelet count <10–$30 \times 10^9/l$)
Initial treatment: see above
Prophylactic treatment: (active patient doing sport, on vacation, etc.)
0.4–0.8 g IVIG/kg body weight once

---

initially). The subsequent treatment procedure depends upon the initial response to IVIG (platelet increase within 72 h, duration of treatment effect). For repetitive treatment in patients with recurrent or chronic ITP at risk for spontaneous bleeding, 0.4 g IVIG/kg body weight given at 2–8-week intervals is recommended, depending on hemorrhagic symptoms. The actual treatment recommendations are summarized in Table 2.

The effect of IVIG was soon confirmed world-wide. A review of 28 published reports[33], including 282 patients, showed that 64% of IVIG-treated individuals had increases in platelet counts above 100×10^9/l, and 83% had increases above 50×10^9/l. Furthermore, after repeated doses of IVIG, splenectomy could be postponed[34]. In adults, Newland[35] documented the existence of two distinct groups with ITP in relation to their response to IVIG treatment. In particular, the response of patients treated early in the course of the disease was different from that of patients treated later. Up to 50% of patients treated within the first 6 months had a long-term response to IVIG alone. Conversely, in virtually all patients treated in the chronic phase (6 months or more after onset of ITP), the response to IVIG was transient. In only occasional adult patients did this author observe prolonged or sustained responses.

ITP and pregnancy

This is a risk for both the fetus and the newborn, since maternal antibodies cross the placenta. Platelets in the baby are eliminated early, i.e. before and within the first few weeks after delivery. The risk of severe ITP ($<50 \times 10^9$/l platelets) is about 20%[36,37]. If a pregnant mother has had a baby with thrombocytopenia in a previous delivery, the new infant is at high risk of bleeding. Fetal platelet counts should be determined by percutaneous umbilical vessel sampling or scalp vein sampling during delivery. If the platelet count is below 50×10^9/l, Cesarean section should be performed[38]. If the platelet count is higher than 50×10^9/l, normal delivery is allowed. The thrombocytopenic infant should be treated by IVIG prophylactically, since the platelet count often continues to decrease within the first few days after birth[39-41]. The recommended dosage of IVIG and the rate of response are the same as in children with acute ITP (Table 2).

Immune neutropenia

In patients with neutropenia, chronic agranulocytosis due to failure of myelopoiesis must be excluded. The autoimmune neutropenia of infancy and early childhood is comparable to ITP in the same age group. Autoimmunity has been documented by neutrophil-specific autoantibodies[42]. IVIG treatment should be limited to the child with increased rates of recurrent infections and skin and/or mucosal alterations due to severe neutropenia (< 500 absolute neutrophil count). Satisfactory responses to IVIG should be evaluated by the diminution of infection rates and the use of antibiotics. The recommended minimal dosage is 0.4 g/kg body weight every 3–4 weeks. In our experience, the response rate with regard to the above-mentioned criteria is over 70%. Others have reported similar response rates using higher doses of IVIG and evaluating the increase of absolute neutrophil count[43]. The response rate is lower in adolescents and adults, and in patients with combined autoimmune disorders.

Autoimmune hemolytic anemia

In patients with autoimmune hemolytic anemia there are only anecdotal reports on the beneficial[44-49] and controversial[49] effects of IVIG treatment. IVIG seems to be less effective and requires higher doses[48] and a longer observation time to evaluate the response. The decrease and normalization of the reticulocyte count is a major criterion of response. We have observed a 6-year-old girl with severe Evan's syndrome who had an unsatisfactory response to corticosteroids, whereas IVIG in a dose of 0.8 g/kg body weight every 3 weeks resulted in complete remission with no hemolytic signs and normalization of the reticulocyte count, despite a continuously positive Coombs reaction. As in other immune cytopenias, such as combined autoimmune anemia with other symptoms/syndromes, IVIG seems to be less effective and it is difficult to form pretreatment estimations of beneficial response. The efficacy of IVIG may differ from individual to individual; on the other hand, IVIG treatment in patients with pure red cell aplasia has led to encouraging results[25,50-52].

FUTURE DIRECTIONS

Future research should be directed towards early recognition of those patients who develop or already have a chronic cytopenia. Determination of antigen–specific autoantibodies may be of diagnostic help. Early treatment with IVIG, together with immunosuppressive agents (corticosteroids, cyclosporin, cyclophosphamide) against cellular pathogenic effects, may postpone the manifestation of chronic disease. In chronic disease the combination of plasmapheresis followed by IVIG replacement should be evaluated.

REFERENCES

1. Harrington, W. J. and Minnich, V. (1951). Demonstration of a thrombocytopenic factor in the blood of patients with thrombocytopenic purpura. *J. Lab. Clin. Med.*, **38**, 1–10
2. Imbach, P., Barandin, S., d'Apuzzo, V. *et al.* (1981). High-dose intravenous γ-globulin for idiopathic thrombocytopenic purpura in childhood. *Lancet*, **1**, 1228
3. Chapman, J. F., Metcalfe, P., Murphy, M. F. *et al.* (1984). Sequential development of platelet, neutrophil and red cell autoantibodies associated with measles infection. *Clin. Lab. Haematol.*, **6**, 219–28
4. Foreman, N. K., Oakhill, A. and Cal, E. O. (1988). Parvovirus associated thrombocytopenic purpura. *Lancet.*, **2**, 1426–7
5. Griffin, D. E., Moench, T. R., Johnson, R. T. *et al.* (1986). Peripheral blood mononuclear cells during natural measles virus infection: cell surface phenotypes and evidence for activation. *Clin. Immunol. Immunopathol.*, **40**, 305–12
6. Shannon, K. M. and Ammann, A. J. (1985). Acquired immune deficiency syndrome in childhood. *J. Pediatr.*, **106**, 332–42
7. ven der Lelle, J., Lange, J. M. A., Vos, J. J. E. *et al.* (1987). Autoimmunity against blood cells in human immunodeficiency virus (HIV) infection. *Br. J. Haematol.*, **67**, 109–14
8. Battaieb, A., Oksenhendler, E., Fromont, P. *et al.* (1989). Immunochemical analysis of platelet autoantibodies in HIV-related thrombocytopenic purpura: a study of 68 patients. *Br. J. Haematol.*, **73**, 241–7
9. Walsh, C. M., Nardi, M. A. and Karpatkin, S. (1984). On the mechanism of thrombocytopenic purpura in sexually active homosexual men. *N. Engl. J. Med.*, **311**, 635–9

10. Karpatkin, S., Nardi, M., Lennette, E. T. *et al.* (1988). Antihuman immunodeficiency virus type 1 antibody complexes on platelets of seropositive thrombocytopenic homosexuals and narcotic addicts. *Proc. Natl. Acad. Sci. USA*, **85**, 9763–7

11. Zon, L. I. and Groopman, J. E. (1988). Haematologic manifestations of the human immune deficiency virus (HIV). *Semin. Hematol.*, **25**, 208–18

12. Klaassen, R. J. L., Mulder, J. W., Viekke, A. B. J. *et al.* (1990). Autoantibodies against peripheral blood cells appear early in HIV infection and their prevalence increases with disease progression. *Clin. Exp. Immunol.*, **81**, 11–17

13. van der Lelie, J., Lange, J. M. A., Goudsmit, J. *et al.* (1989). Idiopathic neutropenia in homosexual men. *Lancet*, **1**, 279

14. Kekomäki, R., Nieminen, U. and Peltolo, H. (1991). Acute idiopathic thrombocytopenic purpura following measles, mumps and rubella vaccination. *Thromb. Haemostas.*, **65**, 866

15. Lane, H. C., Masur, H., Edgar, L. C. *et al.* (1983). Abnormalities of B-cell activation and immunoregulation in patients with the acquired immunodeficiency syndrome. *N. Engl. J. Med.*, **309**, 453–8

16. Rhodes, G., Rumpold, H., Kurki, P. *et al.* (1987). Autoantibodies in infectious mononucleosis have specificity for the glycine–alanine repeating region of the Epstein–Barr virus nuclear antigen. *J. Exp. Med.*, **165**, 1026–40

17. Sumimoto, S., Kasajima, Y., Hamamoto, T. *et al.* (1990). Agranulocytosis following infectious mononucleosis. *Eur. J. Pediatr.*, **149**, 691–4

18. Fujinami, R. S., Nelson, J. A., Walker, L. *et al.* (1988). Sequence homology and immunologic cross-reactivity of human cytomegalovirus with HLA-DR β chain: a means for graft rejection and immunosuppression. *J. Virol.*, **62**, 100–5

19. Young, N. and Mortimer, P. (1984). Viruses and bone marrow failure. *Blood*, **63**, 729–37

20. Sing, G. K. and Ruscetti, F. W. (1990). Preferential suppression of myelopoiesis in normal human bone marrow cells after *in vitro* challenge with human cytomegalovirus. *Blood*, **75**, 1965–73

21. Young, N. (1988). Hematologic and hematopoietic consequences of B19 parvovirus infection. *Semin. Hematol.*, **25**, 159–72

22. Hanada, T., Koike, K., Takeya, T. *et al.* (1988). Human parvovirus B19-induced transient pancytopenia in a child with hereditary spherocytosis. *Br. J. Haematol.*, **70**, 113–15

23. Lefrère, J. J., Courouce, A. M. and Kaplan, C. (1989). Parvovirus and idiopathic thrombocytopenic purpura. *Lancet*, **1**, 279

24. Anderson, L. J. and Török, T. J. (1989). Human parvovirus B19. *N. Engl. J. Med.*, **321**, 536–8

25. Kurtzman, G., Frickhofen, N., Kimbali, J. *et al.* (1989). Pure red-cell aplasia of 10 years' duration due to persistent parvovirus B19 infection and its cure with immunoglobulin therapy. *N. Engl. J. Med.*, **321**, 519–23

26. McMillan, R., Tani, P., Millard, F. *et al.* (1987). Platelet-associated and plasma antiglycoprotein autoantibodies in chronic ITP. *Blood*, **70**, 1040–5

27. Kiefel, V., Santoso, S., Weisheit, M. and Mueller-Eckhardt, C. (1987). Monoclonal antibody-specific immobilization of platelet antigens (MAIPA): a new tool for the identification of platelet-reactive antibodies. *Blood*, **70**, 1722–6

28. Tani, P., Berchtold, P. and McMillan, R. (1989). Autoantibodies in chronic ITP. *Blut*, **59**, 44–6

29. Imbach, P., Tani, P., McMillan, R. *et al.* (1991). Different forms of chronic ITP in children defined by antiplatelet autoantibodies. *J. Pediatr.*, **118**, 535–9

30. Dwyer, J. M. (1992). Manipulating the immune system with immune globulin. *N. Engl. J. Med.*, **326**, 107–16

31. Imbach, P., Wagner, H. P., Berchtold, W. *et al.* (1985). Intravenous immunoglobulin versus oral corticosteroids in acute immune thrombocytopenic purpura in childhood. *Lancet*, **2**, 464–8

32. Imholz, B., Imbach, P., Baumgartner, C. *et al.* (1988). Intravenous immunoglobulin (i.v. IgG) for previously treated acute or for chronic idiopathic thrombocytopenic purpura (ITP) in childhood: a prospective multicenter study. *Blut*, **56**, 63–8

33. Bussel, J. P. and Pham, L. C. (1987). Intravenous treatment with γ-globulin in adults with immune thrombocytopenic purpura: review of the literature. *Vox Sang.*, **52**, 206–11

34. Bussel, J. P., Schulmann, I. Hilgartner, M. W. and Barandun, S.(1983). Intravenous use of γ-globulin in the treatment of chronic immune thrombocytopenia as a means to deter splenectomy. *J. Pediatr.*, **103**, 652–4

35. Newland, A. C. (1986). Clinical and therapeutic aspects and treatment with IV IgG. In Imbach P. (ed.) *Idiopathic Thrombocytopenia: Proceedings of a Workshop*, pp. 63–72. (Bern:Pharmanual, Pharmalibri.)

36. Kelton, J. G., Inwood, M. J., Barr, R. M. *et al.* (1982). The prenatal prediction of thrombocytopenia in infants of mothers with clinically diagnosed immune thrombocytopenia. *Am. J. Obstet. Gynecol.*, **144**, 449–54

37. Samuels, P., Bussel, J. B., Braitman, L. E. *et al.* (1990). Estimation of the risk of thrombocytopenia in the offspring of pregnant women with presumed immune thrombocytopenic purpura. *N. Engl. J. Med.*, **323**, 229–35

38. Martin, J. N., Morrison, J. C. and Files, J. C. (1984). Autoimmune thrombocytopenic purpura: current concepts and recommended practices. *Am. J. Obstet. Gynecol.*, **150**, 86–96

39. Kelton, J. G. (1983). Management of the pregnant patient with idiopathic thrombocytopenic purpura. *Ann. Intern. Med.*, **99**, 796–800

40. Ballin, A., Andrew, M., Ling, E. *et al.* (1988). High-dose intravenous γ-globulin therapy for neonatal autoimmune thrombocytopenia. *J. Pediatr.*, **112**, 789–92

41. Newland, A. C., Boots, M. A. and Patterson, K. G. (1984). Intravenous IgG for autoimmune thrombocytopenia in pregnancy. *N. Engl. J. Med.*, **310**, 261–2

42. Lalezari, P., Khorshidi, M. and Petrosova, M. (1986). Autoimmune neutropenia of infancy. *J. Pediatr.*, **109**, 764–9

43. Bussel, J., Lalezari, P. and Fikrig, S. (1988). Intravenous treatment with γ-globulin of autoimmune neutropenia of infancy. *J. Pediatr.*, **112**, 298–301

44. MacIntyre, E. A., Linch, D. C., Macey, M. G. *et al.* (1985). Successful response to intravenous immunoglobulin in autoimmune hemolytic anemia. *Br. J. Hematol.*, **60**, 387–8

45. Oda, H., Honda, A., Sugita, K. *et al.* (1985). High-dose intravenous intact IgG infusion in refractory autoimmune hemolytic anemia (Evans syndrome). *J. Pediatr.*, **107**, 744–6

46. Pocecco, M., Ventura, A., Tamaro, P. *et al.* (1986). High dose IV IgG in autoimmune hemolytic anemia. *J. Pediatr.*, **109**, 726

47. Besa, E. C. (1988). Rapid transient reversal of anemia and long-term effects of maintenance intravenous immunoglobulin for autoimmune hemolytic anemia in patients with lymphoproliferative disorders. *Am. J. Med.*, **84**, 691–8

48. Bussel, J., Cunningham-Rundles, C. and Abraham, C. (1986). Intravenous treatment of autoimmune hemolytic anemia with very high dose γ-globulin. *Vox Sang.*, **51**, 264–9

49. Mueller-Eckhardt, C., Salama, A., Mahn, I. *et al.* (1985). Lack of efficacy of high-dose intravenous immunoglobulin in autoimmune haemolytic anaemia: a clue to its mechanism. *Scand. J. Haematol.*, **34**, 394–400

50. Clauvel, J. P., Vainchenker, W., Herrera, A. *et al.* (1983). Treatment of pure red cell aplasia by high dose intravenous immunoglobulins. *Br. J. Haematol.*, **55**, 380–1

51. Etzioni, A., Atias, D., Pollack, S. *et al.* (1986). Complete recovery of pure red cell aplasia by intramuscular γ-globulin therapy in a child with hypoparathyroidism. *Am. J. Hematol.*, **22**, 409–14

52. McGuire, W. A., Yang, H. H., Bruno, E. *et al.* (1987). Treatment of antibody-mediated pure red-cell aplasia with high-dose intravenous γ-globulin. *N. Engl. J. Med.*, **317**, 1004–8

13

Intravenous immunoglobulin for the treatment of recurrent pregnancy loss

C. B. Coulam

INTRODUCTION

Recurrent spontaneous abortion is a significant health problem affecting 2–5% of reproducing couples[1]. Although genetic, anatomical and hormonal factors have been implicated in the etiology of recurrent spontaneous abortion, a substantial proportion remain unexplained[2]. An immunological cause has been suggested for more than 80% of otherwise unexplained recurrent spontaneous abortions[3]. Immunotherapy using white blood cells has been proposed as a treatment for these couples[4]. The efficacy of this treatment has been controversial, with some studies reporting beneficial effects[4] and others showing no beneficial effect when compared to placebo-controlled treatments[5,6]. Because of this controversy, alternative treatments for recurrent spontaneous abortion have been sought. Among those reported to result in successful pregnancies is intravenous immunoglobulin (IVIG) therapy[7-15], but none of the studies reporting successful pregnancies after such treatment included control subjects. We therefore undertook a prospective randomized placebo-controlled clinical trial to define the efficacy of IVIG in the treatment of recurrent spontaneous abortion.

MATERIALS AND METHODS

Patients

Women experiencing two or more consecutive spontaneous abortions with the same partner were offered the opportunity of participating in an Institutional Review Board (IRB)-approved randomized placebo-controlled trial using intravenous γ-globulin (IVIG) or albumin (placebo). The obstetric history of each of the women was obtained and the number of total pregnancies, live births, stillbirths, abortions, ectopic pregnancies and hydatidiform moles, and the number of partners, were recorded for each pregnancy. All couples were investigated with chromosome analysis, hysterosalpingography and hysteroscopy, luteal-phase endometrial biopsy and serum progesterone timed with ovulation documented by ultrasonic monitoring of folliculogenesis, anticardiolipin antibody (ACA), activated partial thromboplastin time, human leukocyte antigen (HLA) typing, and assays of the maternal serum for the presence of both complement-dependent and -independent antipaternal antibodies using lymphocytotoxicity assays and mixed lymphocyte culture reactions. All couples with a diagnosis of chromosomal, anatomical, endocrinological and autoimmunological etiology of recurrent pregnancy loss were excluded from the study. Also excluded were women younger than 18 years' or older than 45 years of age, and women with a history of IgA deficiency or hypersensitivity to immunoglobulin. Each woman had blood screened for the presence of human immunodeficiency virus antibodies and hepatitis B antigen.

Sample size consideration

The major determinant of sample size for this type of study is the expected proportion of subsequent pregnancies to end in a spontaneous abortion among the non-intervened group. Estimates provided in the literature suggest 40% as a reasonable expected proportion of third and fourth spontaneous abortions[16]. The next major consideration is the level of reduction to be achieved by the intervention (therapy). If the causes of recurrent spontaneous abortion differ from the causes of isolated spontaneous abortions and can be eliminated by the intervention, the baseline risk for subsequent abortion would be about 12%[16]. Thus, the maximum effect of the treatment would be a decrease in risk of abortion from 0.40 to 0.12, or a 70% reduction. Using traditional parameters for such sample size computations – a type 1 error of 0.05, a type 2 of 0.2 and a one-sided test – 45 pregnancies would be required in the treated and untreated groups.

Protocol

A total of 90 pregnancies were randomized, one half receiving intravenous immunoglobulin (Sandoglobulin®, Sandoz) and the remaining 50% receiving albumin infusions. Each patient receives an intravenous infusion in the follicular phase of the cycle when pregnancy is desired. Patients are randomized to receive either Sandoglobulin® 500 mg/kg per month, or albumin in an intravenous infusion. The patient receives the infusion every 28 days until pregnant, or for 4 months. If the patient is not pregnant in 4 months she is dropped from the study and replaced with another patient. Once conception occurs, the patient receives an infusion every 28 days until delivery, or until 28–32 weeks of gestation.

RESULTS

Figure 1 summarizes the ongoing results of the prospective randomized placebo-controlled trial. To date, 73 women have been enrolled in the study. Study medication has been discontinued in 24 women (34%) who failed to conceive within four cycles after IVIG infusion. Seven women are trying to conceive and 42 women have achieved pregnancies. The outcomes of the 42 pregnancies include ten deliveries, 13 ongoing pregnancies and 19 pregnancy losses.

Of the 19 pregnancy losses, seven (37%) occurred after infusion with IVIG and 12 (63%) after placebo ($p = 0.08$). Ultrasonic examinations of the 19 pregnancy losses revealed seven empty gestational sacs (blighted ova) and 12 intrauterine fetal deaths (fetal pole present with no fetal cardiac activity). Of seven blighted ova, six (86%) were in women receiving IVIG and one (14%) was receiving placebo. Twelve pregnancies ended with intrauterine fetal deaths; 11 (92%) in women receiving placebo and one (8%) in a woman receiving IVIG. Of seven

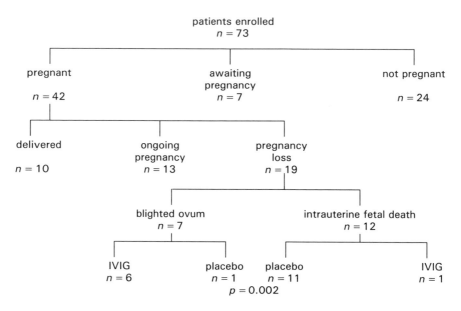

Figure 1 Summary of patients enrolled to date in prospective randomized placebo-controlled clinical trial using intravenous immunoglobulin (IVIG)

pregnancy losses occurring in women receiving IVIG, six (86%) were blighted ova and one (14%) was an intrauterine fetal death. Twelve pregnancy losses occurred in women receiving placebo: one (8%) was a blighted ovum and 11 (92%) were intrauterine fetal deaths. The differences in frequency of blighted ova between IVIG and placebo-treated women was significant ($p = 0.002$).

DISCUSSION

Analysis of an update of the ongoing randomized placebo-controlled clinical trial suggests that IVIG may be efficacious in the treatment of recurrent spontaneous abortion.

IVIG therapy has been previously reported to be effective in the prevention of recurrent spontaneous abortion[7-15], but the mechanism of this antiabortive effect is not known. Immunomodulation by IVIG has been speculated to result from passively transferred blocking or anti–idiotypic antibodies[17], blockade of Fc receptors[18], enhancement of

146

suppressor T-cell function[19], down-regulation of B-cell function[20] and/or reduction of activation of complement components[15,21,22].

Whatever the mode of action, the mechanism does not maintain abnormal pregnancies. The majority of pregnancies lost after treatment with IVIG are blighted ova (Figure 1). Limited data in the literature suggest that the ultrasonic demonstration of an empty sac is associated with an abnormal chromosome analysis of the chorion after chorionic villus sampling[23,24]. If these observations can be confirmed in women experiencing recurrent pregnancy loss, then pregnancies lost after IVIG will be those with abnormal chromosome complements. By contrast, only 8% of pregnancies lost after placebo treatment were associated with a blighted ovum. These preliminary results suggest that IVIG may be successful in maintaining pregnancies not associated with blighted ova and/or abnormal karyotypes. Analysis of data from the completed randomized placebo-controlled trial will test this suggestion.

REFERENCES

1. Coulam, C. B. (1991). Unification of immunotherapy protocols. *Am. J. Reprod. Immunol.*, **25**, 1–6
2. Coulam, C. B. (1986). Unexplained recurrent pregnancy loss: epilogue. *Clin. Obstet. Gynecol.* , **29**, 999–1004
3. McIntyre, J. A., Coulam, C. B. and Faulk, W. P. (1989). Recurrent spontaneous abortion. *Am. J. Reprod. Immunol.*, **21**, 100–4
4. Mowbray, J. E., Lidlee, H., Underwood, J. L. *et al.* (1985). Controlled trial of treatment of recurrent spontaneous abortion by immunization with paternal cells. *Lancet*, **1**, 941–9
5. Ho, H. N., Gill, T. J. III, Hsuish, H. J., Jiang, J. J., Lee, T. Y. and Hsish, C. Y. (1991). Immunotherapy for recurrent spontaneous abortion in a Chinese population. *Am. J. Reprod. Immunol.*, **25**, 10–15
6. Cauchi, M. N., Lemi, D., Young, D. E., Klosa, M. and Pepperell, R. J. (1991). Treatment of recurrent spontaneous aborters by immunization with paternal cells – controlled trial. *Am. J. Reprod. Immunol.*, **25**, 16–17
7. Coulam, C. B., Peters, A. J., McIntyre, J. A. and Faulk, W. P. (1990). The use of intravenous immunoglobulin for the treatment of recurrent spontaneous abortion. *Am. J. Reprod. Immunol.*, **22**, 78

8. Mueller-Eckhardt, O., Heine, G., Neppert, J., Kunzel, W. and Mueller-Eckhardt, C. (1989). Prevention of recurrent spontaneous abortion by intravenous immunoglobulin. *Vox Sang.*, **56**, 151–4

9. Mueller-Eckhardt, G., Huni, O. and Poltrin, B. (1991). IVIG to prevent recurrent spontaneous abortion. *Lancet*, **1**, 424

10. Bernstein, R. M. and Crawford, R. J. (1988). Intravenous IgG therapy for anticardiolipin syndrome: a case report. *Clin. Exp. Rheumatol.*, **6**, 198 (Abstract No. 8)

11. Scott, J. R., Branch, D. W., Kochenour, N. K. and Ward, K. (1988). Intravenous immunoglobulin treatment of pregnant patients with recurrent pregnancy loss caused by antiphospholipid antibodies and Rh immunization. *Am. J. Obstet. Gynecol.*, **159**, 1055–6

12. Carreras, L. Q., Perez, G. N., Vega, H. R. and Casavilla, F. (1988). Lupus anticoagulant and recurrent fetal loss: successful treatment with gammaglobulin. *Lancet*, **2**, 393–4

13. Francois, A., Freund, M., Daffos, F., Remy, P., Riach, M. and Jacquot, C. (1988). Repeated fetal losses and the lupus anticoagulant. *Ann. Intern. Med.*, **109**, 993–4

14. Parke, A., Maier, D., Wilson, D., Andreoli, J. and Ballow, M. (1989). Intravenous γ-globulin, antiphospholipid antibodies and pregnancy. *Ann. Intern. Med.*, **110**, 495–6

15. Christiansen, O. B., Mathiesen, O., Lauristen, J. G. and Grunnet, N. (1992). Intravenous immunoglobulin treatment of women with multiple miscarriages. *Hum. Reprod.*, **7**, 718–22

16. Roman, E. (1984). Fetal loss rates and their relationship to pregnancy order. *J. Epidemiol. Commun. Health*, **38**, 29–35

17. Brand, A., Witvliet, M., Claas, F. H. J. *et al.* (1988). Beneficial effect of intravenous γ-globulin in a patient with complement-mediated autoimmune thrombocytopenia due to IgM-antiplatelet antibodies. *Br. J. Haematol.*, **69**, 507–11

18. Kimberly, R. P., Salmon, J. E., Bussel, J. B. *et al.* (1987). Modulation of mononuclear phagocyte function by intravenous γ-globulin. *J. Immunol.*, **132**, 745–50

19. Delfraissy, J. F., Tchernia, G., Laurian, Y. *et al.* (1985). Suppressor cell function after intravenous γ-globulin treatment in adult chronic idiopathic thrombocytopenic purpura. *Br. J. Haematol.*, **60**, 315–22

20. Nydegger, U. E. (1991). Hypothetic and established action mechanisms of therapy with immunoglobulin G. In Imbach, P. (ed.) *Immunotherapy with Intravenous Immunoglobulins*, pp. 27–36. (London:Academic Press)

21. Kulics, J., Rajnavolgye, E., Fust, G. and Gergely, J. (1983). Interaction of C3 and C3b with immunoglobulin G. *Mol. Immunol.*, **20**, 805–10

22. Zielinski, C. C., Pries, P. and Eibl, M. M. (1985). Effect of immuno-globulin substitution on serum immunoglobulin and complement concentration. *Nephron*, **40**, 253–4

23. Johnson, M. P., Drugan, A., Koppitch, F. C., Uhlmann, W. R. and Evans, M. I. (1990). Postmortem chorionic villus sampling is a better method for cytogenetic evaluation of early fetal loss than culture of abortus material. *Am. J. Obstet. Gynecol.*, **163**, 1505–10

24. Sorokin, Y., Johnson, M. P., Uhlmann, W. R., Zador, I. E., Drugan, A., Koppitch, F. C., Moody, J. and Evans, M. I. (1991). Postmortem chorionic villus sampling: correlation of cytogenetic and ultrasound findings. *Am. J. Med. Genet.*, **39**, 314–16

14

The use of intravenous immunoglobulins in bone marrow transplantation

M. A. Boogaerts

INTRODUCTION

During the past 20 years, bone marrow transplantation (BMT) has progressed from an experimental therapy reserved for end-stage, refractory or relapsed patients, to a therapy of choice for many patients with leukemia, lymphoma, aplastic anemia, myelodysplasia and certain genetic disorders. A number of factors have contributed to these successes in curing diseases of the bone marrow and the immune system[1]: i.e. the study of genetic structures that regulate human tissue type; the development of complex chemoradiotherapeutic regimens that allow destruction of residual malignant cells; the availability of powerful immunosuppressive regimens that allow compatible marrow cells to engraft; and the development of efficient supportive care measures to prevent or control the complications of BMT. Recently, the availability of biological response modifiers and of highly purified intravenous immunoglobulin (IVIG) preparations has greatly improved the prospects for successful BMT outcomes.

High doses of intravenous immunoglobulins have been advocated not only in the prophylaxis of viral (i.e. cytomegalovirus (CMV)) and gram-negative bacterial infections, but also as efficient therapeutic adjuncts and as immunomodulators of graft versus host disease (GVHD)[2,3].

IMMUNODEFICIENCY OF BONE MARROW TRANSPLANTATION

The immune competence of marrow recipients varies during the peritransplant period, depending on the type of host defense mechanisms that are deficient. Each phase of BMT – pretransplant, early post-transplant, mid-recovery and late post-transplant – confers its own risks for infectious complications[1].

Pretransplant period (day −14 to day 0)

The pretransplant conditioning regimen usually damages the skin and mucous membranes, leaving the patient vulnerable to invasion by colonizing gram-positive flora, herpes or candida. The insertion of long-term indwelling central venous catheters can provoke local or systemic infections with staphylococci or other microorganisms. Most transplant centers use elaborate programs for infections, antibiotic and antifungal decontamination, leukocyte-depleted blood products, early empirical antibiotic therapy, and mostly also high-dose IVIG.

Early post-transplant period (day 0 to day +30)

This period is the most dangerous time for infectious complications, because mucosal and skin damage is now accompanied by severe neutropenia, immunosuppressive drugs are used for the prophylaxis and treatment of GVHD, and the first signs of graft failure may become apparent. Both gram-negative and gram-positive bacterial infections may be encountered, but candida and aspergillus remain the most frequently isolated pathogens in the early post-transplant stage. Herpes simplex may lead to mucocutaneous infections, but also to herpes pneumonia, encephalitis and enteritis. The respiratory syncytial virus has increasingly been implicated in viral pneumonia in the early post-transplant stage. Most prophylactic anti-infective protocols will include the administration of high-dose IVIG in this period.

Mid-recovery period (day + 30 to day + 100)

The severe combined immunodeficiency that is the hallmark of the mid-recovery period leads to the predominance of viral rather than bacterial and fungal infections. CMV used to be a major cause of post-BMT mortality, second only to GVHD. Recently, the incidence and mortality of CMV infections has declined due to improved prophylaxis (e.g. IVIG) and more effective therapeutic regimens (e.g. ganciclovir).

Adenovirus and BK-viruses of the papovavirus family have been implicated in the pathogenesis of late-onset hemorrhagic cystitis in this period. Epstein–Barr (EBV) virus infections may induce systemic symptoms such as fever, hepatitis and lymphadenopathy, but can in rare circumstances also terminate in EBV-related lymphoproliferative disease.

Hepatitis C and other hepatitis viruses may be responsible for severe liver function disturbances. Hepatitis may be difficult to distinguish from veno-occlusive disease.

Although bacterial and fungal infections will become less preponderant during the mid-recovery period, care has to be given to *Pneumocystis carinii* prophylaxis, the latter agent being responsible for 10–20% of interstitial pneumonias during this period.

High doses of IVIG have proved their efficacy, especially in this mid-recovery period, more specifically in the prevention of CMV disease.

Late post-transplant period (day + 100 to + 12 months)

Cellular and humoral immune performance will gradually improve during the late post-transplant period, except when chronic GVHD is present and immunosuppressive treatment must continue. Varicella zoster virus infections become more prominent, but life-threatening dissemination is rare. Typically, pneumoccocal (encapsulated) bacteremias are reported in the late recuperation phase of BMT, and may be related to IgG subclass deficiencies. Vaccination can be helpful. Continued high-dose IVIG is indicated for patients with chronic GHVD and hypogammaglobulinemia.

INTRAVENOUS ADMINISTRATION OF IMMUNOGLOBULINS IN BMT

Although the administration of high doses of IVIG has been proven to be beneficial for preventing infections in severely immunocompromised patients, the way it works is still unclear[4]. Direct antiviral, antimicrobial, antifungal and immunomodulatory effects have been implicated. Despite many years of experience with polyspecific IVIG, the appropriate dosages and treatment intervals have not clearly been established[5]. The number of controlled studies is relatively small, and major differences are noted between patient characteristics and types of conditioning regimens, between prophylactic measures for GVHD and between other supportive care measures such as transfusion products and antiviral drugs.

Many investigators have advocated passive immunotherapy with monospecific hyperimmune globulins as opposed to polyspecific preparations[6,7]. The relative efficacy of these different preparations remains difficult to determine while there is no standardization of the various IVIG preparations available, with respect to concentration of antibodies to clinically relevant pathogenic organisms. As a consequence, the variation in antibody content between monospecific and polyspecific preparations (e.g. for anti-CMV antibodies) may be minimal.

Quality control of 59 different lots of Sandoglobulin® (Sandoz) revealed major variations in specific antibody contents. Expressing one standard deviation as a percentage of the mean, antibody activity against diphtheria varied by 67%; against poliomyelitis by 30%; against hepatitis B surface antigen by 35%; against hepatitis A virus by 22%; against measles by 18%; against CMV by 19%; and against anti-streptolysin by 28%[5].

In an intriguing study, 19 antiparvovirus titers out of 25 commercially available IVIG preparations were found to vary between 1/100 and 1/10 000[8].

Therefore, definite recommendations cannot at present be made with regard to the use of one or the other commercially available preparation. All preparations are roughly equivalent in efficacy, safety and ease of administration. Sandoglobulin® (Sandoz) may be better tolerated, whereas Gammagard® (Baxter) may be preferable for IgA-sensitized patients[3,9]

Prophylactic use of IVIG in BMT

Early studies on the use of high–dose immunoglobulins in bone marrow transplantation focused mainly on the prevention of CMV infections or pneumonia[10,11]. The administration of hyperimmune anti–CMV globulin seemed to be very effective in preventing CMV pneumonia in CMV–seronegative patients[12-15]. However, hyperimmune globulin did not protect seronegative patients who received seropositive blood products or bone marrow. In another controlled study of seropositive patients, Rigden and colleagues[16] reported that CMV infection or pneumonia was not prevented by the administration of hyperimmune plasma. Also, in some of these early studies, the incidence of interstitial pneumonia from all causes, and even of septicemia, seemed to be lower[17,18]. The overall survival rate and incidence of acute GVHD seemed not to be influenced by hyperimmune IVIG.

CMV prophylaxis with commercially available polyspecific IVIG preparations proved to be equally effective as with the monospecific products. Symptomatic CMV infections developed in significantly fewer seronegative patients treated post–BMT with either 0.5 g/kg every 14 days until 120 days post–transplant, or with 1.0 g/kg given weekly until 120 days post–transplant[14,15].

In the studies with polyspecific immunoglobulins, trends were noted towards lower incidences of acute and chronic GVHD but no influence was seen on the development of other viral, bacterial or fungal infections.

An impressive study on the immunomodulatory and antimicrobial efficacy of IVIG in BMT was published by Sullivan and colleagues[19]. A total of 382 patients were enrolled, including those with CMV seropositivity, advanced age and disease status and human leukocyte antigen (HLA)–non-identical marrow donors. Patients randomized to IVIG (500 mg/kg weekly from day 7 to day 90, then monthly to day 360 post-transplant) were compared to controls not given IVIG. Among 61 evaluable seronegative patients transfused with CMV–seronegative blood products, none developed interstitial pneumonia. Among 308 seropositive patients, 22% of controls and 13% of IVIG recipients developed interstitial pneumonia. Control patients had an increased relative risk of gram–negative septicemia and local infection, and received considerably more units of platelets than did IVIG recipients. In patients over 20 years of age the incidence of acute GVHD was reduced. Consequently, a decrease in deaths due to transplant-related causes after transplantation of HLA-identical marrow was noted. The favorable results of this study must be interpreted with caution, however, because neither overall survival nor the risk of relapse was altered by IVIG. The latter may be related to the fact that high doses of IVIG have the potential to attenuate the graft versus leukemia effect associated with GVHD[20].

The antimicrobial and antiviral properties of IVIG probably rely on mere antibody replacement, enhanced neutralization and clearance, augmented opsonophagocytic function, improved complement activation and more efficient antibody-dependent cellular cytotoxity[19].

The immunomodulatory effects are more complex, and depend mostly on the class (IgG versus IgM) as well as the idiotypic determinates of the immunoglobulin molecule[21]. IVIG may also interfere with the activity of many of the cytokines that are involved in inflammatory processes and GVHD[22]. Moreover, this immunomodulatory effect may have much to do with the intimate relationship which exists between GVHD and infection in allogeneic BMT. Since relatively germ-free patients develop less severe GVHD[23], effective prevention of infections may result in a reduction of GVHD incidence. Also, viral infection has been implicated in the facilitation of GVHD, possibly via an increased expression of HLA molecules. Further arguments for immunomodulation by IVIG can be found in the fact that immunoglobulin treatment has been effective in the treatment of numerous autoimmune disorders, possibly through interference with cellular immune functions[24,25] (e.g. inhibition of overall T-cell activation or augmented T-cell suppressor activity, restriction of B-cell differentiation or anti-idiotypic regulation)[26,27].

The effects of IVIG on platelet half-life are thought to depend on saturating macrophage Fc receptors[28]. Increased serum IgG levels might therefore be related to rates of platelet consumption. In a recent study by Cottler-Fox and co-workers[29], IgG levels were monitored after the infusion of standard doses of IVIG. High IgG trough levels (> 1200 mg/dl) were associated with fewer platelet transfusions and showed a trend towards a decreased incidence of sepsis. However, low serum IgG trough levels (< 1200 mg/dl) appeared to be strongly associated with acute GVHD. Pharmacokinetic modeling revealed a shorter IgG half-life (i.e. increased utilization) in the immediate peritransplant period (day -8 to day $+6$) for those allogeneic recipients who developed acute GVHD. This altered half-life of IVIG may reflect an intrinsic difference between transplant recipients which predisposes to acute GVHD and low IgG trough levels. The authors concluded that it may become possible to predict in advance which recipients are at increased risk of acute GVHD, and that prophylaxis might be optimized on an individual basis[30].

Following the reports[31,32] of improved survival in established CMV pneumonia in BMT patients following combined therapy with high-dose IVIG and ganciclovir, trials were initiated on the prophylactic use of this combination. This approach may be beneficial, especially in CMV-seropositive patients. Yau[33] has shown that, using this combined approach, the incidence of interstitial pneumonitis and the cumulative probability of CMV excretion in the first 100 days post-transplant was significantly reduced.

THERAPEUTIC USE OF IVIG IN BMT

Not many studies have been published on the therapeutic use of IVIG in BMT patients[34,35]. Although a certain degree of consensus may exist on the dose and scheduling of prophylactic IVIG, appropriate dosages for therapeutic use are unknown. Optimal scheduling of combinations with artivirals, antibiotics or antifungals is largely empiric[36].

In conjunction with antibiotics, intravenous immunoglobulins decrease the mortality due to sepsis in premature infants weighing less than 1500 g whose immune systems are very similar to those of BMT patients[3,37,38].

Intravenous immunoglobulins have also been used in the treatment of HIV-infected children when their antibody-forming capacity is severely compromised (low IgG levels) or when infectious syndromes (e.g. sinusitis or diarrhea) persist despite optimal antibiotic therapy.

In BMT the combination of high-dose IVIG and ganciclovir has been shown to be effective in the treatment of established CMV pneumonia. 'Pre-emptive' therapy (i.e. starting upon detection of the virus in excreta or bronchoalveolar lavage via early antibody or antigen tests) with high-dose immunoglobulins with or without ganciclovir, can avoid the development of invasive CMV disease[39,40]. Recently, the use of IVIG has also been advocated in the treatment of parvovirus B19 infections post-BMT[41].

In analogy to studies performed in severely septic surgical patients[42], high-dose IVIG may prove to be beneficial in the treatment of sepsis and multiple organ failure in BMT patients. However, monoclonal antibodies may be more efficient in the bacterial setting. In a multicenter randomized double-blind study, a monoclonal antilipid A IgM antibody, administered to patients with demonstrated gram-negative bacteremia, improved survival in both bacteremic and septic shock patients[43]. Also, IgM- and IgA-enriched intravenous immunoglobulin preparations have been postulated to exert major antiendotoxin properties, thereby possibly leading to better survival in gram-negative bacteremia[21]. Although endotoxin is an important stimulator of cytokine production (e.g. interleukin-1, interleukin-6, tumor necrosis factor), antiendotoxin antibodies may also lead to immunomodulation of inflammatory responses and graft versus host (GVH) reactions.

Finally, it should be stressed that therapeutic doses of IVIG have also been shown to improve the response to single donor platelets in patients refractory to pooled platelet transfusions, and to ameliorate post-BMT autoimmune cytopenia[28]. Delayed hypogammaglobulinemia or immunoglobulin subclass deficiencies (e.g. IgG2 and IgG4) post-BMT may be adequately corrected by IVIG[9,34].

SIDE-EFFECTS OF INTRAVENOUS IMMUNOGLOBULINS IN BMT

The administration of high-dose IVIG has become standard practice in both the prophylaxis and the treatment of viral and bacterial infections in BMT. This has much to do not only with the reported positive effects, but also with the overall safety of the commercially available preparations[9]. The new pH 4.25 preparations can be infused in large amounts, with few vasomotor symptoms or other toxicities. Chills, fever, flushing, headache, pruritus, nausea or myalgia are occasionally observed, but may continue for several hours. Slowing the rate of infusion, prior treatment with paracetamol or antihistamines, or temporary interruption of the infusion may be efficient counter-measures. Corticosteroids are seldom necessary. Severe anaphylactic reactions are rare, and are mostly related to selective IgA deficiency with antibodies to IgA in the recipient[44]. Classic therapy with epinephrine, steroids, oxygen and antihistamines is indicated. Gamma-gard contains very low concentrations of IgA and can be safely given to IgA-deficient, IgA-antibody-positive patients, under careful supervision.

The transmission of viral agents has not been described with modern IVIG preparations, with the possible exception of a few hepatitis non-A, non-B cases[37,45] and a late aseptic meningitis case[46].

Hyperviscosity and renal insufficiency have been reported with very high doses of IVIG, or in dehydrated patients[47]. Fluid overload may lead to transient pulmonary edema, but this can easily be prevented by furosemide prophylaxis in patients at risk.

The immunomodulatory effects of high-dose IVIG should not be underestimated[48]. A definite risk of alloimmunization exists, resulting in a serum sickness-like syndrome. Intravascular hemolysis may be caused by the presence of hemagglutinins in many products[49].

High-dose IVIG has been implicated in the impairment of endogenous antibody formation[50] (negative feedback). In patients with systemic vasculitis, treated by IVIG, a 51% decrease in antineutrophil cytoplasm antibodies was noted[51]. T-cell activation[52] and natural killer cell activity[53] may be inhibited, which may have much to do with the alleged role of high-dose prophylactic IVIG in the abro-gation of GVH, but also of graft versus leukemia reactions. Anti-idiotypic antibodies, present in the commercially available IVIG preparations, may impair B-cell development[54,55], whereas blockade of the Fc receptor may interfere with the normal clearance of other infectious agents and with the normal process of opsonophagocytosis. An alternative approach to this problem is the use of monoclonal antibodies.

A common problem encountered with the use of high-dose IVIG in the early post-transplant period resides in the unreliability of serological diagnosis of infectious diseases. False-positive results may be obtained due to passive transfer of antibodies[26].

The long-term side-effects have not been documented. However, aseptic meningitis has been recorded[46].

PROSPECTS FOR THE FUTURE

Whereas the regular use of IVIG in the prophylaxis and treatment of infections post-BMT has become generally accepted, some newer pathways are increasingly explored:

(1) The use of cocktails of monoclonal antibodies or IgM-enriched preparations[2,21];

(2) The use of combinations of IVIG and antiviral drugs (ganciclovir)[56];

(3) The use of combinations of IVIG and biological response modifiers (e.g. growth factors)[26]; and

(4) The use of specific B-cell differentiation agents (e.g. B-cell colony-stimulating factor, IL-7, etc.)[26].

In the meantime there is great need for further studies defining adequate dosages, schedules and intervals[57], 'best' preparations and pharmacodynamics (half-life)[58] in BMT patients.

Not much is known about the long-term effectiveness of passive immunotherapy. The incidence of late infections and of chronic GHVD during continued long-term administration of IVIG has so far not specifically been studied.

CONCLUSIONS

Because of its overall safety, IVIG has increasingly been used for the prophylaxis and treatment of various infections in the peritransplant period. However, the precise indications and potential hazards should carefully be delineated.

If properly used, the currently available IVIG preparations allow for better and safer anti-infective supportive care in the early post-transplant period. As such, IVIG has a definite place in the therapeutic armamentarium of BMT protocols. Optimal dosages range between 0.5 and 1.0 g/kg, with intervals from weekly to fortnightly, starting 7 days before the procedure and continuing for at least 4-6 months post-transplant. If longer use is envisaged, the high cost of these preparations should be taken into consideration.

REFERENCES

1. Boogaerts, M. A. (1992). Bone marrow transplantation. In *Current Concepts*, pp. 3–44. (Kalamazoo:Scope Publications)
2. Nydegger, U. E. (1992). Intravenous immunoglobulin in combination with other prophylactic and therapeutic measures. *Transfusion*, **32**, 72–82
3. Stiehm, E. R. (1991). New uses for intravenous immunoglobulins. *N. Engl. J. Med.*, **325**, 123–5
4. Sullivan, K. M. (1987). Immunoglobulin therapy in bone marrow transplantation. *Am. J. Med.*, **83** (Suppl. 4), 34–45
5. Nydegger, U. E. (1992). Clinical relevance of optimal versus maximal doses of prophylactic and therapeutic immunoglobulins. In Dominioni, L. and Nydesser, U. E. (eds.) *Immunoglobulins Today and Tomorrow*, pp. 11–25. (London:Royal Society of Medicine Services)
6. Chehimi, J., Peppard, J. and Emmanuel, D. (1987). Selection of an intravenous immune globulin for the immunoprophylaxis of cytomegalovirus infections: an *in vitro* comparison of currently available and previously effective immune globulins. *Bone Marrow Transplant.*, **2**, 395–402
7. Winston, D. J., Pollard, R. B., Ho, W. G., Gallagher, J. G., Rasmussen, L. E., Huang, N. S., Lin, C. H., Gossett, T. G., Merigan, T. C. and Gale, R. P. (1982). Cytomegalovirus immune plasma in bone marrow transplant recipients. *Ann. Int. Med.*, **97**, 11–18
8. Schwarz, T. F., Roggendorf, M., Hottenträger, B., Modrow, S., Deinhardt, F. and Middendorp, J. (1990). Immunoglobulins in the prophylaxis of parvovirus B19 infection. *J. Inf. Dis.*, **162**, 1214–15
9. Buckley, R. H. and Schiff, R. I. (1991). The use of intravenous immunoglobulin in immunodeficiency diseases. *N. Engl. J. Med.*, **325**, 110–17
10. Condie, R. M. and O'Reilly, R. J. (1984). Prevention of cytomegalovirus infection by prophylaxis with an intravenous, hyperimmune, native unmodified cytomegalovirus globulin. Randomized trial in bone marrow transplant recipients. *Am. J. Med.*, **76** (Suppl. 3A), 134–41
11. Kubanek, B., Ernst, P., Ostendorf, P., Schafer, U. and Wolf, H. (1985). Preliminary data of a controlled trial of intravenous hyperimmune globulin in the prevention of cytomegalovirus infection in bone marrow transplant recipients. *Transplant Proc.*, **17**, 468–9
12. Meyers, J. D., Leszczynski, J., Zaia, J. A., Flournoy, N., Newton, B., Snydman, D. R., Wright, G. G., Levin, M. J. and Thomas, E. D. (1983). Prevention of cytomegalovirus infection by cytomegalovirus immune globulin after marrow transplantation. *Ann. Intern. Med.*, **98**, 442–6
13. O'Reilly, R. J., Reich, L., Gold, J., Kirkpatrick, D., Dinsmore, R., Kapour, N. and Condie, R. (1983). A randomized trial of intravenous hyperimmune

globulin for the prevention of cytomegalovirus (CMV) infections following marrow transplantation: preliminary results. *Transplant Proc.*, **15**, 1405–11

14. VuVan, H., Fieere, D., Chomel, J., Thonvenot, D., Guyotat, D., Duton, L., Ginestet, C., Lacroze, M. and Aymard, M. (1985). Prophylaxis against cytomegalovirus infection after BMT with gammaglobulins. (Abstr.) *Exp. Hematol.*, **13** (Suppl. 17), 105

15. Winston, D. J., Ho, W. G., Lin, C-H., Bartoni, K., Budinger, M. D., Gale, R. P. and Champlin, R. E. (1987). Intravenous immune globulin for prevention of cytomegalovirus infection and interstitial pneumonia after BMT. *Ann. Intern. Med.*, **106**, 12–18

16. Rigden, O., Pilhstedt, P., Volin, L., Nikoskelainen, J., Lonnquist, B., Ruutu, P., Ruutu, T., Toivanen, A. and Wahren, B. (1987). Failure to prevent cytomegalovirus infection by cytomegalovirus hyperimmune plasma: a randomized trial by the Nordic Bone Marrow Transplantation Group. *Bone Marrow Transplant.*, **2**, 299–305

17. Graham-Pole, J., Camitta, B., Casper, J., Elfenbein, G., Gross, S., Herzig, R., Koch, P., Mahony, D., Marens, R. and Munoz, L. (1988). Intravenous immunoglobulin may lessen all forms of infection in patients receiving allogeneic BMT for acute lymphoblastic leukemia: a pediatric oncology group study. *Bone Marrow Transplant.*, **3**, 559–66

18. Petersen, F., Bowden, R., Thornquist, M., Meyers, J. D., Buckner, C. D., Counts, G. W., Nelson, N., Mewton, B. A., Sullivan, K. M. and Melver, J. (1987). The effect of prophylactic intravenous immunoglobulins on the incidence of septicemia in marrow transplant recipients. *Bone Marrow Transplantation*, **2**, 141–8

19. Sullivan, K. M., Kopecky, K. J., Jacom, J., Fisher, L., *et al.* (1990). Immunomodulatory and antimicrobial efficacy of intravenous immunoglobulin in BMT. *N. Engl. J. Med.*, **323**, 705–12

20. Sullivan, K. M., Storb, R., Buckner, C. D., Fefer, A., Fisher, L., Weiden, P. L., Witherspoon, R. P., Appelbaum, F. R., Banaji, M. and Hansen, J. (1989). Graft-versus-host disease as adoptive immunotherapy in patients with advanced hematologic neoplasms. *N. Engl. J. Med.*, **320**, 828–34

21. Poynton, C. H., Jackson, S., Fegan, C., Barnes, R. A. and Whittaker, J. A. (1992). Use of IgM enriched intravenous immunoglobulin (Pentaglobin) in bone marrow transplantation. *Bone Marrow Transplant.*, **9**, 451–7

22. Cohen, J. (1988). Cytokines as mediators of graft-versus-host disease. *Bone Marrow Transplant.*, **3**, 193–7

23. Van Bekkum, D. W. and Knaan, S. (1977). Role of bacterial microflora in development of intestinal lesions from graft-versus-host reaction. *J. Natl. Cancer Inst.*, **58**, 787–90

24. Bussel, J., Pahwa, S., Porges, A., Cunningham-Rundles, S., Koziner, B., Morell, A. and Barandum, S. (1986). Correlation of *in vitro* antibody synthesis with the outcome of intravenous gammaglobulin treatment of chronic idiopathic thrombocytopenic purpura. *J. Clin. Immunol.*, **6**, 50–6

25. Delfraissy, J. F., Tchernia, G., Laurian, Y., Wallon, C., Galanaud, P. and Dormont, J. (1985). Suppressor cell function after intravenous gamma-globulin treatment in adult chronic idiopathic thrombocyopenic purpura. *Br. J. Haematol.*, **60**, 315–22

26. Storek, J. and Saxon, A. (1992). Reconstitution of B cell immunity following bone marrow transplantation. *Bone Marrow Transplant.*, **9**, 395–408

27. Sultan, Y., Kazatchkine, M. D., Maisonneuve, P. and Nydegger, V. E. (1984). Anti-idiotypic suppression of autoantibodies to factor VIII (anti-haemophilic factor) by high-dose intravenous gammaglobulin. *Lancet*, **2**, 765–8

28. Zeigler, Z. R., Shadduck, R. K. and Rosenfeld, C. S. (1987). High-dose intravenous gamma-globulin improves responses to single-donor platelets in patients refractory to platelet transfusion. *Blood*, **70**, 1433–6

29. Cottler-Fox, M., Lynch, M., Pickle, L. W., Cahill, R., Spitzer, T. R. and Deeg, H. J. (1991). Some but not all benefits of intravenous immunoglobulin therapy after marrow transplantation appear to correlate with IgG trough levels. *Bone Marrow Transplant.*, **8**, 27–33

30. Schiff, R. I. (1985). Individualizing the dose of intravenous immune serum globulin for therapy of patients with primary humoral immunodeficiency. *Vox Sang.*, **49** (Suppl.1), 15–24

31. Emmanuel, D., Cunningham, J., Jules-Elysee, K., Brochstein, J. A., Kernan, N. A., Laver, J., Stover, D., White, D. A., Fels, A., Polsky, B., Castro-Malaspina, H., Peppard, J. R., Bartus, P., Hammerling, U. and O'Reilly, R. J. (1988). Cytomegalovirus pneumonia after bone marrow transplantation successfully treated with the combination of ganciclovir and high-dose intravenous immune globulin. *Ann. Intern. Med.*, **109**, 777–82

32. Lehn, P. (1990). Treatment of severe cytomegalovirus infection with ganciclovir and high-dose intravenous immunoglobulins in patients with allogeneic bone marrow transplantation. *Nouv. Rec. Fr. Hematol.*, **32**, 17–20

33. Yau, J. C. (1991). Prophylaxis of cytomegalovirus infection with ganciclovir in allogeneic bone marrow transplantation. *Eur. J. Hematol.*, **47**, 371–6

34. N.I.H. Consensus Development Conference (1990). Intravenous immunoglobulins, prevention and treatment of disease. *J. Am. Med. Assoc.*, **264**, 3189–93

35. Snydman, D. R. (1990). Cytomegalovirus immunoglobulins in the prevention and treatment of cytomegalovirus disease. *Rev. Infect. Dis.*, **12**, S838–S847

36. Winston, D. J. (1987). Intravenous immunoglobulins as therapeutic agents: use in viral infections. *Ann. Intern. Med.*, **107**, 371–4

37. Björkander, J., Cunningham-Rundles, C., Lundin, P., Olsson, R., Söderström, R. and Hanson, L. Å. (1988). Intravenous immunoglobulin prophylaxis causing liver damage in 16 of 77 patients with hypogammaglobulinemia or IgG subclass deficiency. *Am. J. Med.*, **84**, 107–11

38. Noya, F. J. D., Rench, M. A., Garcia-Prats, J. A., Jones, T. M. and Baker, C. J. (1988). Disposition of an immunoglobulin intravenous preparation in very low birth weight neonates. *J. Pediatr.*, **112**, 278–83

39. Reed, E. C., Bowden, R. A., Dandliker, P. S., Lilleby, K. E. and Meyers, J. D. (1988). Treatment of CMV pneumonia with ganciclovir and intravenous CMV Ig in patients with BMT. *Ann. Intern. Med.*, **109**, 783–8

40. Verdonck, L. F., de Gast, G. C., Dekker, A. W., de Weger, R. A., Schuurman, H. J. and Rozenberg-Arska, M. (1989). Treatment of CMV pneumonia after BMT with CMV Ig combined with ganciclovir. *Bone Marrow Transplant*, **4**, 187–9

41. Kurtzman, G., Frickhofen, N., Kimball, J., Jenkins, D. W., Nienhuis, A. W. and Young N. S. (1989). Pure red-cell aplasia of 10 years' duration due to persistent parvovirus B19 infection and its cure with immunoglobulin therapy. *N. Engl. J. Med.*, **321**, 519–23

42. Dominioni, L., Dionigi, R. and Zanello, M. (1991). Effects of high dose IgG on survival of surgical patients with sepsis score of 20 or greater. *Arch. Surg.*, **126**, 236–40

43. Ziegler, E. J., Fisher, C. J. and Sprung, C. L. (1991). Treatment of gram-negative bacteremia and septic shock with a HA-1A human monoclonal antibody against endotoxin. *N. Engl. J. Med.*, **324**, 429–36

44. Burks, A. W., Sampson, H. A. and Buckley, R. H. (1986). Anaphylactic reactions after gammaglobulin administration in patients with hypogammaglobulinemia: detection of IgE antibodies to IgA. *N. Engl. J. Med.*, **314**, 560–4

45. Weiland, O., Mattsson, L. and Glaumann, H. (1986). Non-A, non-B hepatitis after intravenous gammaglobulin. *Lancet*, **1**, 976–7

46. Casteels-Van Daele, M., Wijndaele, L., Hunninck, K., and Gillis, P. (1990). Intravenous immune globulin and acute aseptic meningitis. *N. Engl. J. Med.*, **323**, 614–15

47. Rault, R., Piraïno, B., Johnston, J. R. and Oral, A. (1991). Pulmonary and renal toxicity of intravenous immunoglobulins. *Clin. Nephrol.*, **36**, 83–8

48. White, W. B., Desbonnet, C. R. and Ballow, M. (1987). Immunoregulatory effects of intravenous serum globulin therapy in common variable hypogammaglobulinemia. *Am. J. Med.*, **83**, 431–6

49. Kim, H. C., Park, C. L., Cowan, J. H., Frattori, F. D. and August, C. S. (1988). Massive intravascular hemolysis associated with IVIg in BMT recipients. *Am. J. Ped. Hem. Onc.*, **10**, 69–74

50. Kawada, K. and Terasaki, P. (1987). Evidence of immunosuppression by high-dose gammaglobulin. *Exp. Hematol.*, **15**, 133–6

51. Jayne, D. R. W., Davies, M. J., Fox, C. J. V., Black, C. M. and Lockwood, C. M. (1991). Treatment of systemic vasculitis with pooled intravenous immunoglobulin. *Lancet*, **337**, 1137–9

52. Durandy, A., Fischer, A. and Griscelli, C. (1981). Dysfunction of pokeweed mitogen-stimulated T and B lymphocyte responses induced by gammaglobulin therapy. *J. Clin. Invest.*, **67**, 867–77

53. Engelhard, D., Waner, J. L., Kapoor, N. and Good, R. A. (1986). Effect of intravenous immune globulin on natural killer cell activity: possible association with autoimmune neutropenia and idiopathic thrombocytopenia. *J. Pediatr.*, **108**, 77–81

54. Hashimoto, F., Sakiyama, Y. and Matsumoto, S. (1986). The suppressive effect of gamma-globulin preparations on *in vitro* pokeweed mitogen-induced immunoglobulin production. *Clin. Exp. Immunol.*, **65**, 409–15

55. Stohl, W. (1986). Cellular mechanisms in the *in vitro* inhibition of pokeweed mitogen-induced B cell differentiation by immunoglobulin for intravenous use. *J. Immunol.*, **136**, 4407–13

56. Schmidt, G. M., Kovacs, A., Zaia, J. A., Horak, D. A., Blume, K. G., Nademanee, A. P., O'Donnell, M. R., Snyder, D. S. and Forman, S. J. (1988). Ganciclovir/immunoglobulin combination therapy for the treatment of human cytomegalovirus-associated interstitial pneumonia in bone marrow allograft recipients. *Transplantation*, **46**, 905–7

57. Gratwohl, A., Doran, J. E., Bachmann, P., Scherz, R., Späth, P., Baumgartner, C., Perret, B., Berger, C., Nissen, C., Tichelli, A., Speck, B. and Morell, A. (1991). Serum concentrations of immunoglobulins and of antibody isotypes in bone marrow transplant recipients treated with high doses of polyspecific immunoglobulin or with cytomegalovirus hyperimmune globulin. *Bone Marrow Transplant.*, **8**, 275–82

58. Rand, K. H., Houck, H., Ganju, A., Babington, R. G. and Elfenbein, G. J. (1989). Pharmacokinetics of cytomegalovirus-specific IgG antibody following intravenous immunoglobulin in bone marrow transplant patients. *Bone Marrow Transplant.*, **4**, 679–83

15

Intravenous immunoglobulin in children with AIDS

M. M. S. Carneiro-Sampaio

Pediatric cases constitute a significant proportion of patients from acquired immune deficiency syndrome (AIDS) nowadays: about 2% of all AIDS reported cases are younger than 15-years-old. The course of the disease in children can be rapid and lethal: the survival time of HIV-infected children is usually shorter than that of adults.

According to the latest official data released by the Brazilian Ministry of Health on 1 August 1992, 29 634 cases of AIDS have been reported in that country. Of these, 969 (3.3%) belong to the pediatric group, most of whom were infected by their own mothers, either perinatally or by vertical transmission. Certainly the main problem of AIDS in Brazil during the last few years has been the sharp increase in the number of infected women. The male : female ratio in 1992 was 6 : 1, whereas until 1988 it was more than 30 : 1. The most common cause of HIV infection among young adult women in Brazil is intravenous drug use.

Unlike adults, pediatric AIDS patients suffer from frequent and sometimes severe bacterial infections, due mainly to encapsulated microorganisms such as *Streptococcus pneumoniae* and *Hemophilus influenzae* (Table 1)[1-3]. Human immunodeficiency virus- (HIV) infected children frequently present with an infection pattern that is similar to that observed in children with primary antibody synthesis disorders. HIV-infected children are prone to extracellular bacterial infections, since their ability to form specific antibodies is severely affected and because they have no previously developed spectrum of antibodies to protect

Table 1 Main AIDS indicator diseases in 3471 cases in children under 12 years of age (Centers for Disease Control, December 31, 1991)[2]

AIDS indicator disease	Cumulative frequency (%)
Pneumocystis pneumonia	38
Lymphoid interstitial pneumonia	25
Recurrent bacterial infections	21
Candida esophagitis	15
Wasting	13
HIV encephalopathy	12

them from pyrogenic as well as viral infections. B-cell dysfunction occurs very early in pediatric AIDS. Although they have impaired antibody production, most pediatric AIDS patients present with elevated serum immunoglobulin levels (Figures 1–4) (Marques and Grumach; Fujimura *et al.*, unpublished observations). Hypergammaglobulinemia usually appears early in HIV-infected infants, and reflects B-cell polyclonal activation. In adult AIDS patients, about 30% of B-cell clones are involved in anti-HIV antibody synthesis[4]; in this sense it is not a typical polyclonal activation but rather an 'oligoclonal' phenomenon.

Between 1986 and 1989, preliminary trials were published on the therapeutic use of intravenous immunoglobulin (IVIG) in pediatric AIDS patients[5-9]. In addition to small numbers of cases, historic or non-randomly selected patients were used as controls. In all studies, IVIG-treated children had fewer infectious episodes and more prolonged survival times, even though the ultimate mortality rate did not alter significantly.

After pilot studies, the National Institute of Child Health and Human Development (NICHHD) in the USA sponsored a large multicenter double-blind placebo-controlled (albumin) study on the use of IVIG to prevent infections in both symptomatic (P2) and asymptomatic but with abnormalities in immune response (P1B) children[10,11]. A total of 372 HIV-infected patients were evaluated. They were under 13 years of age, without hemophilia, and were stratified into two groups according to CD4+ lymphocyte count at the entry into the study as well as by

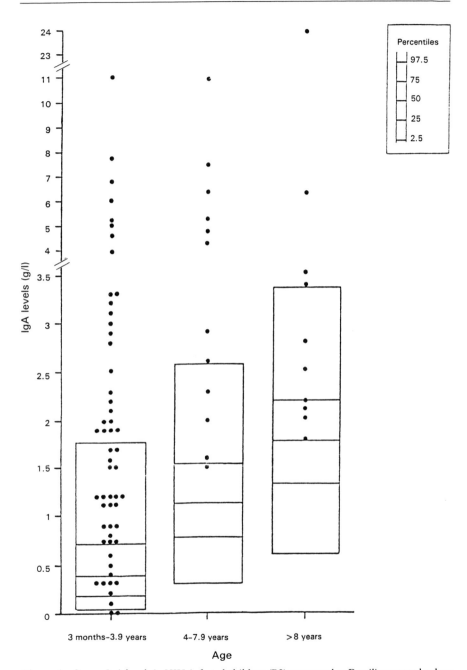

Figure 1 Serum IgA levels in HIV-infected children (P2) compared to Brazilian normal values

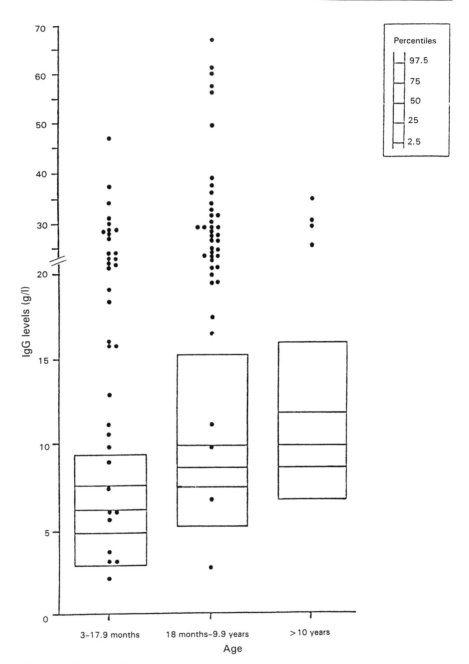

Figure 2 Serum IgG levels in HIV-infected children (P2) compared to Brazilian normal values

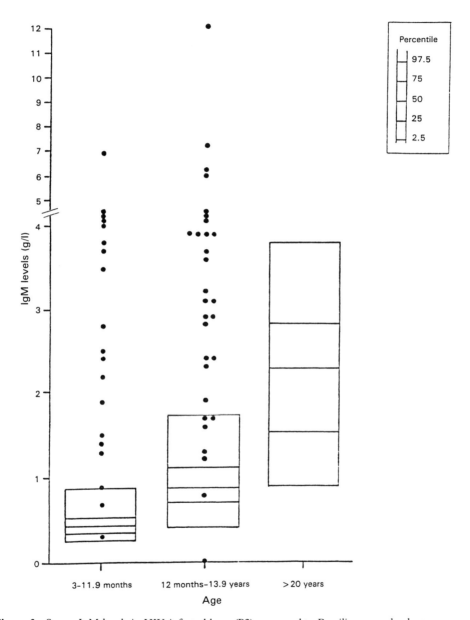

Figure 3 Serum IgM levels in HIV-infected boys (P2) compared to Brazilian normal values

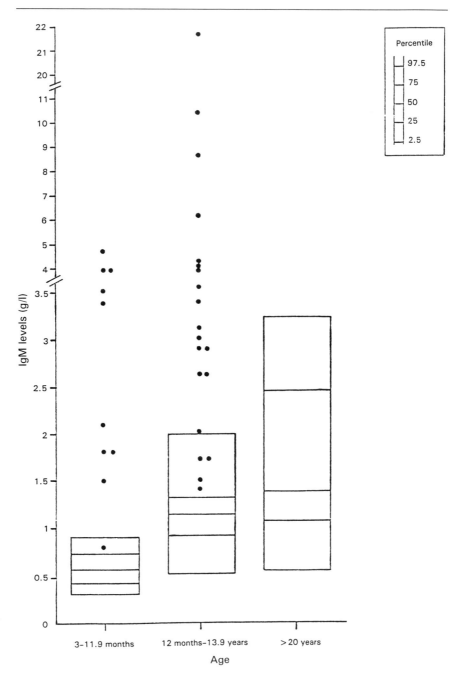

Figure 4 Serum IgM levels in HIV-infected girls (P2) compared to Brazilian normal values

Centers of Disease Control, USA (CDC) clinical classification. Patients received 400 mg/kg body weight each 28 days, and the median length of follow-up was 17 months; 39% began zidovudine (AZT) therapy after entry into the study, whereas 49% were receiving *Pneumocystis carinii* prophylaxis by the end of the trial.

The conclusions of this study are that the prophylactic use of IVIG is safe, since adverse reactions were observed in less than 1% of cases. The treatment significantly increased the number of periods free from serious bacterial infection, significantly reduced the number of both serious and minor bacterial infections, and significantly decreased the numbers of hospitalizations for acute care in those patients who entered treatment with CD4+ counts higher than 200 cells/mm^3. However, mortality was not affected in any group of CD4+ count at entry.

From these encouraging results, it can be seen that IVIG is clearly indicated in HIV-infected children, and it must be introduced early in the course of the infection.

The use of IVIG in the management of adults with AIDS is not justified, since no real benefits have been observed, according to case reports and trials published to date.

The possible mechanisms of action of IVIG in HIV-infected children are as follows[12]:

(1) As replacement therapy for patients who present with severe impairment of antibody synthesis, as noted previously. This is probably the main mechanism by which IVIG favors the clinical course of AIDS in children.

(2) As immunomodulation therapy. Some clinical trials with IVIG have shown that treatment can improve HIV-associated immunodepression. Such observations include stabilization or even an increase in helper T-lymphocyte counts, an improvement in lymphocyte proliferative mitogenic response, the removal of circulating immune complexes, and a decrease in dehydrogenase values[7,8].

(3) As an attempt to suppress autoimmune reactions. The role of autoimmunity in the pathogenesis of pediatric AIDS has not so far been well evaluated. In adults, autoimmune reactions are associated with a variety of clinical manifestations, such as renal dysfunction, severe neurological disorders, and especially with hematological

findings. Thrombocytopenic purpura is a common finding in pediatric HIV infection, and high doses of IVIG have been recommended to treat these cases[1,13]. Platelet aggregation induced by circulating immune complexes (platelets as innocent bystanders) seem to be important mechanisms in the pathogenesis of thrombocytopenia in HIV-infected patients.

In conclusion, the available data clearly indicate that IVIG must be used in symptomatic HIV-infected children, and also in those who are asymptomatic but who have an alteration in their immune response (P1B)[10,14,15]. Clinical trials using IVIG associated with zidovudine and prophylaxis for *P. carinii* are currently being conducted, including one co-ordinated by NICHHD, and the results are eagerly expected.

ACKNOWLEDGEMENT

I am indebted to Dr Heloisa Helena de Souza Marques from Instituto da Criança 'Professor Pedro de Alcantara' who kindly allowed me to present her data about serum immunoglobulin levels.

REFERENCES

1. Carneiro-Sampaio, M. M. S., Grumach, A. S., Marques, H. H. S., Duarte, A. S. S. and Oselka, G. W. (1988). Caraterísticas Clínicas e laboratóriais de crianças com SIDA. *Cadernos de Imuno-Alergologia Pediátrica*, **3**, 5–13
2. Hanson, I. C. (1993). Respiratory infections in HIV-infected children. *Immunol. Clin. N. Am.*, **13**, 205–17
3. Falloon, J., Eddyr, J., Wiener, L. and Pizzo, P. (1989). Human immunodeficiency virus infection in children. *J. Pediatr.*, **144**, 1–30
4. Amadori, A., De Rossi, A., Faulkner-Valle, G. P. and Chieco-Bianchi, L. (1988). Spontaneous *in vitro* production of virus-specific antibody by lymphocytes from HIV-infected subjects. *Clin. Immunol. Immunopathol.*, **46**, 342–51
5. Calvelli, T. A. and Rubinstein, A. (1986). Intravenous γ-globulin in infant acquired immunodeficiency syndrome. *Pediatr. Infect. Dis.*, **5**, S207–S210
6. Silverman, B. A. and Rubinstein, A. (1985). Serum lactate dehydrogenase levels in adults and children with acquired immune deficiency syndrome

(AIDS) and AIDS-related complex: possible indicator of B-cell lymphoproliferation and disease activity. Effect of intravenous γ-globulin on enzyme levels. *Am. J. Med.*, **78**, 728–36

7. Grupta, A., Novick, B. E. and Rubinstein, A. (1986). Restoration of suppressor T-cell functions in children with AIDS following intravenous γ-globulin treatment. *Am. J. Dis. Child.*, **140**, 143–6

8. Wood, C. C., McNamara, J. G., Schwartz, D. F., Merrill, W. W. and Shapiro, E. D. (1987). Prevention of pneumococcal bacteremia in a child with acquired immunodeficiency syndrome–related complex. *Pediatr. Infect. Dis.*, **6**, 564–6

9. Hague, R. A., Yap, P. L., Mok, J. Y. Q. *et al.* (1989). Intravenous immunoglobulin in HIV infection: evidence for the efficacy of treatment. *Arch. Dis. Child.*, **64**, 1146–50

10. National Institute of Child Health and Human Development Intravenous Immunoglobulin Study Group (1991). Intravenous immune globulin for the prevention of bacterial infections in children with symptomatic human immunodeficiency virus infection. *N. Engl. J. Med.*, **325**, 73–80

11. Centers for Disease Control (1987). Classification system for human immunodeficiency virus (HIV) infection in children under 13 years of age. *MMWR*, **35**, 225–35

12. Schaad, U. B. (1992). IVIG in the management of HIV infection in children. In Dominioni, L. and Nydegger, U. E. (eds.) *Intravenous Immunoglobulins: Today and Tomorrow*, pp. 51–5. (London:Royal Society of Medicine Services)

13. Ellaurie, M., Burns, E. R., Bernstein, L. J., Shah, K. and Rubinstein, A. (1988). Thrombocytopenia and human immunodeficiency virus in children. *Paediatrician*, **82**, 905–8

14. Buckley, R. H. and Schiff, R. I. (1991). Drug therapy: the use of intravenous immune globulin in immunodeficiency diseases. *N. Engl. J. Med.*, **325**, 110–18

15. Stiehm, E. R. (1991). New uses for intravenous immune globulin. *N. Engl. J. Med.*, **325**, 123–5

16

Treatment of juvenile rheumatoid arthritis with high doses of intravenous γ-globulin

B. González Martín

Juvenile rheumatoid arthritis (JRA) is a heterogeneous group of diseases that affect young people under 16 years of age, and the diagnosis is based on clinical criteria as well as on evolutional changes. Laboratory tests play an important role when assigning patients to the different clinical varieties proposed by the American Rheumatological Academy (ARA).

One variety of JRA is systemic arthritis, whose main clinical manifestations are fever, adenopathy, arthritis and morbilliform rash. This variety constitutes 20% of all the JRA cases we have assessed in the last 10 years. The outcome of the illness is uncertain, and some young patients need high and steady doses of corticosteroids to check the condition. As a consequence of these treatments patients often suffer serious complications and severe growth retardation. For these reasons we thought it interesting to analyze the impact of treatment with intravenous γ-globulin (Sandoglobulin®, Sandoz) in patients suffering from the systemic variety of JRA, assessing the effect of the treatment on the general symptoms, corticosteroid consumption and the eventual immunological changes that this immunomodulating therapy could have.

We selected five children aged 2–14 years (mean = 7.2 years) suffering from systemic JRA, diagnosed according to the criteria established by the ARA, and who were clinically active at the start of the present study. All of them had been treated with non-steroidal anti-inflammatory drugs and then with prednisolone, with no evident results. Previous follow-up time varied from 0.9 to 9 years, with an average of 3.14

years. Intravenous γ-globulin (400 mg kg^{-1} day^{-1}) was given for 3 consecutive days[1,2]. The results showed an important clinical improvement in three children, who had a reduction in the CD4/CD8 ratio (-44.7%) with an increment in the CD8 subpopulations ($+195\%$). Two patients who did not show any improvement had an increment in the CD4/CD8 ratio due to a diminution of CD8 subpopulations (-40.5%).

These preliminary results suggest that γ-globulin could benefit patients suffering from JRA of the systemic variety. Monitoring of T-cell subpopulations, specially the increment of CD8, could be an immunological indicator of the immunomodulating activity of this preparation.

REFERENCES

1. Groothoff, J. and Van Leeuwen, E. F. (1988). High-dose intravenous γ-globulin in chronic systemic juvenile arthritis. *Br. Med. J.*, **296**, 1362
2. Mitropoulu, J., Becker, H. and Helmke, K. (1987). High-dose intravenous immunoglobulins in rheumatoid arthritis. *Clin. Exp. Rheumatol.*, **5**, 205

17

Intravenous γ-globulin: an alternative treatment in severe steroid-dependent asthma

E. W. Gelfand and B. D. Mazer

INTRODUCTION

Concern over the increasing morbidity, rate of hospitalization and even mortality of asthma has stimulated a reassessment of the approaches to its treatment[1,2]. Increasing emphasis has been placed on the role of inflammation in asthma, and the need for medications to better control the inflammatory responses which contribute to bronchoconstriction. However, despite optimal treatment with inhaled cromolyn or corticosteroids, certain patients require systemic corticosteroid therapy[3]. These patients are therefore at risk for significant adverse side-effects, including growth suppression, weight gain, Cushingoid features, hypertension, cataracts and spontaneous bone fractures.

In the hope of relieving the need for systemic corticosteroid therapy, alternative therapies have been considered. These have been directed to increasing the effectiveness of corticosteroids (e.g. troleandomycin) or reducing inflammation (e.g. gold, methotrexate, dapsone). These alternative therapies also carry the potential risk of further adverse effects, and often necessitate long-term treatment[4-8].

Intravenous γ-globulin (IVIG) has been used effectively in the treatment of humoral immune deficiencies[9]. It is a safe preparation with no long-term side-effects. Its use in autoimmune disorders began in the early 1950s, with the treatment of immune thrombocytopenic purpura[10]. More recently, IVIG has reportedly been successful in the treatment of a wide variety of autoimmune cytopenias, anti-factor VIII associated coagulopathy, myasthenia gravis and antineutrophil cytoplasmic antigen (ANCA)-associated systemic vasculitis[11-13]. The mode of action of IVIG in these disorders has not been clarified, but theories include Fc receptor blockade of reticuloendothelial system macrophages[14], the provision of anti-idiotypic antibodies[15], or immunomodulation, possibly by inducing CD8+ suppressor T cells[16].

IVIG AS AN ANTI-INFLAMMATORY AGENT

Although the mechanism of action of IVIG is not clear, there is increasing evidence that it may have potent anti-inflammatory activity. In patients with polymyositis[17] or systemic juvenile rheumatoid arthritis[18], the major benefit of IVIG appears to be in the reduction of inflammation, as noted by the changes in erythrocyte sedimentation rate, fever, rash and lymphadenopathy. The beneficial effects of IVIG in Guillain-Barré syndrome or chronic inflammatory demyelinating polyneuropathy may also reside in the anti-inflammatory action of the drug[19]. The most obvious demonstration of this anti-inflammatory activity has been observed in the IVIG treatment of Kawasaki disease[20]. In addition to the prevention of coronary artery abnormalities, infusions of IVIG have a remarkably rapid effect on a number of acute inflammatory parameters[21]. These responses include a reduction in fever, granulocyte count and acute-phase reactants (e.g. C-reactive protein, α_1-antitrypsin). Importantly, the reduction of inflammation seen with IVIG in this diverse array of diseases has provided opportunities to reduce the use of corticosteroids or cytotoxic drugs.

RATIONALE FOR USING IVIG IN ASTHMA

Since it has been established that asthma is an inflammatory disease, and that IVIG has anti-inflammatory activities, it was logical to consider the use of IVIG in the treatment of severe steroid-dependent asthma. There are also additional considerations supporting the potential for IVIG in asthma. Several observations suggest that IgE and/or allergens contribute to the pathogenesis of asthma. Epidemiological studies by Burrows and colleagues[22] and Sears and co-workers[23] demonstrated a close correlation between serum IgE levels and the propensity to develop asthma. Experimental allergen-challenge reactions in the skin and airways of atopic individuals are generally characterized by an IgE-dependent biphasic reaction[24]. Within minutes of exposure to an allergen, mast cells bearing IgE directed to the relevant allergen become activated and release mediators, chemotactic factors and cytokines. This immediate reaction is classically evident within 15–60 min of challenge, and subsides 30–90 min later. After 3–12 h there often develops an intense inflammatory reaction, termed the late-phase reaction (LPR), characterized by the infiltration and activation of esosinophils, neutrophils and mononuclear cells. Increasingly, the IgE-mediated LPR is thought to play an important role in the pathogenesis of chronic allergic diseases.

There are a number of mechanisms by which IVIG may modulate IgE-mediated responses: first, it may inhibit the differentiation of B cells to antibody-secreting cells after stimulation[25]. IVIG may therefore act in a non–isotype-specific manner to decrease IgE synthesis; second, allergen-specific IgG present in IVIG may bind to allergens, blocking their interaction with cell-bound IgE – so-called 'blocking antibodies'; third, IVIG may act by decreasing target organ (cell) sensitivity to the allergen; and fourth, IVIG may down-regulate allergen-specific IgE responses by providing a source of anti-idiotypic antibodies. Anti-idiotypic antibodies have been shown to be present in commercial IVIG preparations[26].

IVIG IN ASTHMA

Study design

An initial open-labelled study was carried out in eight children[27] ranging from 6 to 17 years of age. An additional patient has been added to the original series. All patients had severe asthma (defined by American Thoracic Society criteria), and had been receiving oral steroid therapy for 1–8 years. Patients averaged more than one exacerbation of their asthma per month during the preceding years, often necessitating short bursts of high-dose oral corticosteroids. Prior to the trial, multiple attempts to decrease their steroid dose were without success. Excluded from the study were patients with a second, complicating respiratory disease, subjects receiving allergen immunotherapy, and patients with abnormal responses to immunization with specific antigens.

IVIG (Sandoglobulin®, Sandoz) was infused as a 6% solution. Each patient received $1\,g\,kg^{-1}\,day^{-1}$ for 2 days every 4 weeks for 6 months. During the initial 2 months prior to IVIG (pre-IVIG) each patient underwent full pulmonary function testing, including body plethysmography. A panel of skin-prick tests to common Colorado antigens was performed. The antigens eliciting the most positive reactions were chosen for repeated testing by end-point titration. Reactions were outlined by felt pen and tape transferred to score sheets. Wheal surface areas were calculated with a program to outline and measure the tape-transferred wheal tracings. Peak expiratory flow rates (PEFR) were measured twice daily, before and after inhaled medication, and logged. Symptom scores, monitored from 0 (no symptoms) to 4 (severe, incapacitating symptoms) were also logged for cough, shortness of breath, chest discomfort, wheezing episodes, medication changes, and numbers of inhaled treatments with β-agonists.

Before each infusion and 4 weeks after the final infusion, symptom scores, PEFR and skin test responses were evaluated. Medication adjustments were based on the patients' clinical status. Statistical analysis was carried out by the Student's t-test for comparison of 'before and after' measures, and analysis of variance was used for any multiple comparisons with a repeated measures analysis.

RESULTS

Steroid requirements

The average alternate-day steroid dosage during the 2-month observation period for the nine patients prior to IVIG therapy was $29.3 \pm 5.5\,mg$ (Table 1). On completion of 6 months of IVIG therapy, the average alternate-day steroid dose was $15.6 \pm 2.5\,mg$, a significant reduction. In addition to the need for a regular intake of corticosteroids, these patients often required pulses of corticosteroids for acute exacerbations of their asthma. As illustrated in Table 1, during the

Table 1 Effect of intravenous immunoglobulin (IVIG) on steroid requirements

	Pre-IVIG★	*IVIG*
Average alternate-day steroid dose (mg)	29.3 ± 5.5	15.6 ± 2.5
Average monthly steroid dose (mg) for asthma exacerbations	164 ± 11	64 ± 3

★ Values are means ± SE for nine patients

evaluation period before IVIG therapy, this group of patients required 164 ± 11 mg of oral steroids monthly for exacerbations, but only 64 ± 3 mg on average for each month while on IVIG.

Peak expiratory flow rates

Monitoring of PEFR revealed two groups of patients. In the first group normal PEFR were maintained but high doses of oral corticosteroids were required (Figure 1(a)). In this group, IVIG permitted a marked reduction in steroid usage, with maintenance of normal PEFR. In the second group (Figure 1(b)), in the face of low doses of oral corti-costeroids, PEFR were abnormally low. However, on IVIG, PEFR results normalized without increasing the need for oral steroids.

Symptom scores

All subjects completed daily symptom diaries rating symptoms from 0 (no symptoms) to 4 (incapacitating symptoms). Figure 2 illustrates that analysis of individual diary symptoms scores, compiled for each 4-week period, revealed a marked improvement while on IVIG. This improve-ment was also accompanied by a 50% decrease in the need for extra treatments of inhaled β-agonists while on IVIG.

Skin-test responses

Of the eight patients initially enrolled in the trial, seven responded to one or more antigens by prick testing. During the course of IVIG

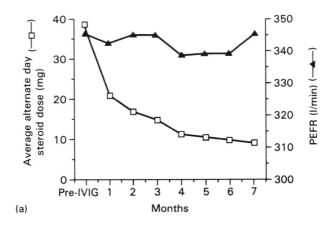

(a)

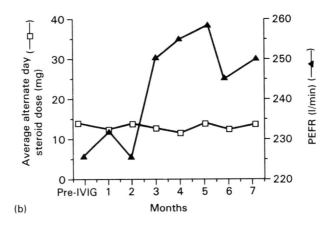

(b)

Figure 1 Effect of intravenous immunoglobulin (IVIG) on peak expiratory flow rates (PEFR). In eight patients, PEFR were continuously monitored on a daily basis and average monthly PEFR are plotted along with average alternate-day steroid dose. Two groups were distinguished: (a) the first group ($n = 5$) required high doses of corticosteroids to maintain normal peak flow rates; (b) the second group ($n = 3$) had low PEFR while maintained on lower doses of the drug

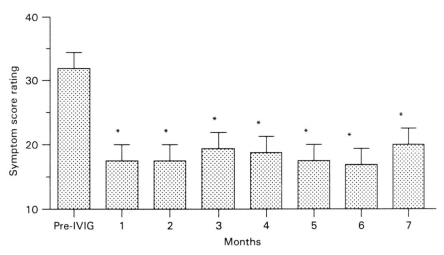

Figure 2 Average monthly symptom scores. Patients maintained a daily diary evaluating symptom scores for six parameters: cough, shortness of breath, chest discomfort, morning wheezing, nocturnal wheezing and wheezing during daytime activities. The average monthly symptom score rating decreased significantly after the first infusion, and was maintained throughout the trial ($p < 0.005$). Values indicated are mean ± SE. IVIG, intravenous immunoglobulin

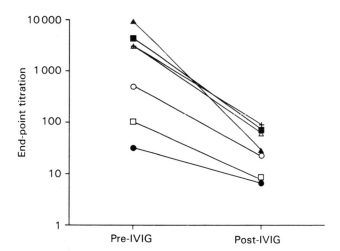

Figure 3 Changes in prick skin-test reactivity. Patients enrolled in the trial were tested monthly with a panel of up to five antigens to which they were sensitive. These antigens were end-point titrated in tenfold dilutions. The average end-point titrations for all antigens in seven patients are illustrated before therapy and 1 month after the last infusion. All patients had a significant decrease in end-point titration. IVIG, intravenous immunoglobulin

therapy, there was a progressive reduction in skin-test reactivity in these individuals. On completion of 6 months of therapy, this decrease in skin-test reactivity was highly significant, averaging a 100-fold decrease in reactivity to each antigen (Figure 3). At the same time, the skin-test responses to histamine were unaffected.

Follow-up

We have now begun to analyze the data in patients who have completed one cycle of IVIG followed by 6 months 'off' IVIG therapy. These preliminary results indicate some deterioration in PEFR after the 6-month period off IVIG, with an increase in average monthly oral corticosteroids needed for exacerbations. In parallel, there was a deterioration in symptom scores. During the 'off' period, there was an increase in skin-test reactivity to known allergens.

CONCLUSIONS

Passive immunity for protection with γ-globulin was initiated in the 1950s for patients with antibody deficiency diseases. What was remarkable in treating these patients was that replacement therapy with γ-globulin had benefits apparently beyond simple infection prophylaxis. Associated with replacement therapy, remission of a number of different skin conditions, including eczema, autoimmune cytopenias, and reactive airway disease, was also seen. These observations suggested that IVIG may have additional benefits in certain autoimmune or allergic disorders. It is becoming increasingly clear that IVIG does indeed have a role in the therapy of a number of diseases currently being treated with corticosteroids and/or cytotoxic drugs. The mechanism of action of IVIG in any of these disorders is not clear, and may reflect immunomodulatory and/or anti-inflammatory effects.

Heightened airways responsiveness is a major feature of asthma. In terms of the mechanisms that initiate these responses, allergen-specific IgE appears to be a major feature of the disease. As a consequence of the interaction of allergen with IgE bound to mast cells, inflammatory mediators and cytokines are released, resulting in the infiltration of the airways with inflammatory cells. Thus, airways hyper-responsiveness can be seen as the outcome of heightened immunological and/or inflammatory responses.

In children with severe steroid-dependent asthma, IVIG, in an open-labelled study, reduced corticosteroid dependency and corticosteroid morbidity without apparent toxicity. Overall, steroid requirements were significantly reduced both in terms of regular intake and the amounts needed to control acute exacerbations. The steroid-sparing effects of IVIG were accompanied by significant improvements in PEFR and symptom scores. The onset of IVIG activity appeared surprisingly rapidly, since the ability to taper steroids, improvements in symptom scores and the increases in PEFR were observed even after the first infusion.

The mechanism of action of IVIG in asthmatic patients is also unclear. Is the benefit related to similar anti-inflammatory effects observed in some collagen-vascular diseases? IVIG has immunomodulatory effects, at least *in vitro*, on mitogen-induced proliferation or immunoglobulin production. Support for an immunomodulatory effect in asthma may be the observed reduction in skin-test reactivity to defined allergens, seen in all patients. The reductions in skin-test reactivity were progressive during the 6-month period of therapy with IVIG, and decreases were also observed after the initial infusion.

It appears that IVIG may provide an alternative therapy for severe asthmatics to minimize the need for systemic corticosteroids, and to reduce the adverse effects of the steroids. This potential for IVIG in asthma must be confirmed in a larger randomized placebo-controlled trial. Further, delineation of the mechanism of action of IVIG is imperative if proper trials are to be initiated and attention paid to dose requirements and frequency of infusions. As in other diseases with prominent immune and inflammatory components, IVIG may provide the severe asthmatic with an option to reduce steroid morbidity and relieve steroid dependency.

REFERENCES

1. Weiss, K. B. and Wagener, D. K. (1990). Changing patterns of asthma mortality. Identifying target populations at high risk. *J. Am. Med. Assoc.*, **264**, 1683–7

2. Gergen, P. J. and Weiss, K. B. (1990). Changing patterns of asthma hospitalization among children: 1979 to 1987. *J. Am. Med. Assoc.*, **264**, 1688–92

3. Barnes, P. J. (1989). New concepts in pathogenesis of bronchial hyper-responsiveness and asthma. *J. Allergy Clin. Immunol.*, **83**, 1013–26

4. Wald, J. A., Friedman, B. F. and Farr, R. S. (1986). An improved protocol for the use of troleandomycin (TAO) in the treatment of steroid-requiring asthma. *J. Allergy Clin. Immunol.*, **78**, 36–43

5. Mullarkey, M. F., Webb, D. R. and Pardee, N. E. (1986). Methotrexate in the treatment of steroid-dependent asthma. *Ann. Allergy*, **56**, 347–50

6. Mullarkey, M. F., Blumenstein, B. A., Andrade, W. P., Barley, G. A., Olason, J. and Wetsel, C. E. (1988). Methotrexate in the treatment of corticosteroid-dependent asthma. A double-blind crossover study. *N. Engl. J. Med.*, **318**, 603–7

7. Muranaka, M., Miyamatoto, T., Shida, T., Kabe, J., Makino, S., Okumura, H., Takeda, K., Suzuki, S., and Horiuchi, Y. (1988). Gold salt in the treatment of bronchial asthma – a double-blind study. *Ann. Allergy*, **40**, 132–7

8. Bernstein, D. I., Bernstein, I. L., Bodenheimer, S. S. and Pietrusko, R. G. (1988). An open study of Auranofin in the treatment of steroid-dependent asthma. *J. Allergy Clin. Immunol.*, **81**, 6–16

9. Buckley, R. H. (1987). Immunodeficiency diseases. *J. Am. Med. Assoc.*, **258**, 2841–9

10. Imbach, P., Barandun, S., d'Apuzzo, V., Baumgartner, C., Hirt, A., Morell, A., Rossi, E., Schöni, M., Vest, M. and Wagner, H. P. (1981). *Lancet*, **1**, 1228–30

11. Khaveri, S. V., Dietrich, G. and Kazatchkine, M. D. (1992). Can intravenous immunoglobulin treatment regulate autoimmune responses? *Semin. Hematol.*, **29**, 64–71

12. Gadjos, P. H., Outin, H., Elkharrat, D., Brunel, D., de Rohan-Chabot, P., Raphael, J. C., Goulon, M., Goulon-Goeau, C. and Morel, E. (1984). *Lancet*, **1**, 406–7

13. Sultan, Y., Kazatchkine, M. D., Maisonneuve, P. and Nydegger, U. E. (1984). Anti-idiotypic suppression of autoantibodies to factor VIII (antihaemophilic factor) by high-dose intravenous gammaglobulin. *Lancet*, **2**, 765–70

14. Fehr, J., Hoffman, V. and Kappelar, V. (1982). Transient reversal of thrombocytopenia in idiopathic thrombocytopenic purpura by high-dose intravenous gamma globlulin. *N. Engl. J. Med.*, **306**, 1254–8

15. Dietrich, G. and Kazatchkine, M. D. (1990). Normal immunoglobulin G (IgG) for therapeutic use (intravenous Ig) contain antiidiotypic specificities against an immunodominant, disease-associated, cross-reactive idiotype of human antithyroglobulin autoantibodies. *J. Clin. Invest.*, **85**, 620–5

16. Tsubakio, T., Kurata, Y., Katagiri, S., Kanakura, Y., Tamaki, T., Kuyama, J., Kanayama, Y., Yonezawa, T. and Tarui, S. (1983). Alternation of T cell subsets and immunoglobulin synthesis *in vitro* during high dose γ-globulin therapy in patients with idiopathic thrombocytopenic purpura. *Clin. Exp. Immunol.*, **53**, 697–702

17. Roifman, C. M., Schaffer, F. M., Wachsmuth, S. G., Murphy, G. and Gelfand, E. W. (1987). Reversal of chronic polymyositis following intravenous immune serum globulin therapy. *J. Am. Med. Assoc.*, **258**, 513–15

18. Silverman, E. D., Laxer, R. M., Greenwald, M., Gelfand, E. W., Shore, A., Stein, L. D. and Roifman, C. M. (1990). Intravenous gamma globulin therapy in systemic juvenile rheumatoid arthritis. *Arthritis Rheumatism*, **33**, 1015–22

19. Vermeulen, M., van der Meche, F. G., Speelman, J. D., Weber, A. and Busch, H. F. (1985). Plasma and gamma-globulin infusion in chronic inflammatory polyneuropathy. *J. Neurol. Sci.*, **70**, 317–26

20. Newburger, J. W., Takahashi, M., Burns, J. C., Beiser, A. S., Chung, K. J., Duffy, C. E., Glode, M. P., Mason, W. H., Reddy, V., Sanders, S. P., Shulman, S. T., Wiggins, J. W., Hicks, R. V., Fulton, D. R., Lewis, A. B., Leung, D. Y. M., Colton, T., Rosen, F. S. and Melish, M. E. (1986). The treatment of Kawasaki syndrome with intravenous gamma globulin. *N. Engl. J. Med.*, **315**, 341–7

21. Leung, D. Y. M. (1989). The immunologic effects of IVIG in Kawasaki disease. *Int. Rev. Immunol.*, **5**, 197–202

22. Burrows, B., Martinez, F. D., Halonen, M., Barbee, R. A. and Cline, M. G. (1989). Association of asthma with serum IgE levels and skin-test reactivity to allergens. *N. Engl. J. Med.*, **320**, 271–7

23. Sears, M. R., Burrows, B., Flannery, E. M., Herbison, G. P., Hewitt, C. J. and Holdaway, M. D. (1991). Relation between airway responsiveness and serum IgE in children with asthma and in apparently normal children. *N. Engl. J. Med.*, **325**, 1067–71

24. Few, A. J. and Kay, A. B. (1990). Eosinophils and T-lymphocytes in late-phase allergic reactions. *J. Allergy Clin. Immunol.*, **85**, 533–9

25. Hashimoto, F., Sakiyama, Y. and Matsumoto, S. (1986). The suppressive effect of gammaglobulin preparation on *in vitro* pokeweed mitogen-induced immunoglobulin production. *Clin. Exp. Immunol.*, **65**, 409–15

26. Rossi, F. and Kazatchkine, M. D. (1989). Antiidiotypes against auto-antibodies in pooled normal human polyspecific Ig. *J. Immunol.*, **143**, 4104–9

27. Mazer, B. D. and Gelfand, E. W. (1991). An open-label study of high-dose intravenous immunoglobulin in severe childhood asthma. *J. Allergy Clin. Immunol.*, **87**, 976–83

18

Immunoglobulins in autoimmune disorders

E. Rewald

We already have an updated idea of the known and speculative mechanisms by which high doses of intravenous immunoglobulins (IVIG) may act in autoimmune disorders. The effects of IVIG on certain inflammatory phenomena have also been discussed. It is my purpose briefly to review the clinical aspects of some autoimmune diseases, emphasizing symptoms such as fever and inflammation (Figure 1), which may be influenced by IVIG, either transitorily or in a sustained fashion. We have seen that autoimmunity is not always limited to the interaction of immunoglobulins and T and B lymphocytes. This may be just the beginning of a complex activation of an ever-increasing amount of powerful substances, released mostly from the cells involved, also including natural killer cells and accessory cells such as macrophages, granulocytes and others. Besides the modulation of synthesis and release of inflammatory mediators, molecular cascades such as those of complement and coagulation may also be activated in the serum.

In acquired hemophilia, the IgG autoantibody that inhibits the procoagulant activity of the factor VIII coagulant complex (FVIII:C) is associated with profuse and often life-threatening hemorrhage. It may occur spontaneously in otherwise healthy individuals, or it may arise in women postpartum, in patients with rheumatoid arthritis (RA), systemic lupus erythematosus (SLE), or drug allergy (e.g. penicillin). These antibodies differ from the alloantibodies to FVIII:C that may be generated by infusion of factor VIII in patients with severe hemophilia. The response to immunosuppressive agents such as prednisone and azathioprine is quite variable. Spontaneous remission may occur with considerable frequency. As has already been discussed elsewhere, Sultan and colleagues[1] have demonstrated the suppression of high-titer FVIII : C inhibitors in two non-hemophilic patients by injecting high doses of IVIG. Since then, IVIG has become a standard therapy for this condition, in spite of some failures[2]. Success with the treatment has also been reported in hemophilia A with alloantibodies to FVIII : C[3], and in hemophilia B with antibodies to factor IX[4]. Moffat and co-workers[5] did not confirm this, as they found no anti-idiotypes to hemophilic alloantibodies in the normal population. We and others[6,7] have observed that in acquired hemophilia treated with high-dose IVIG, the hemorrhagic tendency seems to disappear even before the factor VIII rises to a functional level.

The use of high-dose IVIG seems also of benefit in acquired von Willebrand syndrome[8]. An acquired von Willebrand factor (vWF) inhibitor has been seen in patients with angiodysplasia, solid tumors or myelodysplastic syndrome. However, its most striking association is with diseases involving the immune system, including systemic lupus erythematosus (SLE), benign monoclonal gammopathies, lympho-proliferative disorders and multiple myeloma. Apart from the immunomodulating action of IVIG, Macik and colleagues[8] speculate that a possible effect on endothelial cells could play a role in a similar fashion to desmopressin acetate, either by stimulating production of vWF or by promoting the release of stores.

Wong and colleagues[9] reported the results of studies conducted by Lian and co-workers which showed that, in thrombotic thrombocyto-penic purpura (TTP), plasma caused the aggregation of both autologous and homologous platelets, which was inhibited by IgG from normal adults. Based on these findings it has been reported that IVIG in combi-nation with plasmapheresis might be advantageous for the treatment of refractory TTP. Nevertheless, the failure rate of IVIG in the treatment of TTP is apparently high[10].

Circulating autoantibodies to neutrophil cytoplasm antigens (ANCA) have been identified in patients with diverse types of systemic vasculitis, such as Wegener's granulomatosis, rheumatoid vasculitis and micro-scopic polyarteritis. Jayne and associates[11] have found anti-idiotypic antibodies in IVIG which react with idiotypes on ANCA, and similar anti-idiotypic antibodies in the serum of postrecovery patients. All seven of their patients responded positively; five went into full remission, one showed sustained improvement, and the other had only a partial, transient recovery. The rise in ANCA during and soon after IVIG therapy was not associated with exacerbation of the disease. The subsequent rate of fall in ANCA suggests inhibition of further antibody synthesis by IVIG. There is a concern that IVIG might exacerbate renal damage, as has been seen in certain cases of lupus nephritis[12], but no adverse effect on serum creatinine was found at follow-up. Kawasaki syndrome, a childhood disease where IVIG has been shown to be particularly successful, has been related to this group of vasculitides. Although its etiology is still unknown, suspicion is strong about the possibility that this self-limited syndrome with characteristic epidemiological features is infectious. Nevertheless, there are also findings that suggest an important alteration of the immunological 'homeostasis' in Kawasaki syndrome. Among the immune abnormalities are ANCA-positivity, a decrease in suppressor CD8 cells and activation of CD4 cells. Besides elevated levels of interleukin-2 (IL-2), the IgM fraction of acute Kawasaki syndrome sera has been shown to be cytolytic to endothelial cells if these are pretreated with interferon-γ (IFN-γ), IL-1, or tumor necrosis factor (TNF)[3]. This inflammatory process over 1–2 weeks concentrates on the perivascular area, but frequently granulocytes (increased oxygen intermediate generation) affect the intima. The coronary arterial walls are a frequent target and, in consequence, Kawasaki syndrome currently exceeds acute rheumatic fever as the leading cause of acquired heart disease in children in the US[13]. In a multicenter controlled trial, Furusho and colleagues[14] demonstrated that the usual high doses of IVIG, in association with aspirin, were of benefit in preventing coronary artery aneurysms, provided that treatment was started early enough (within 7 days of onset of fever). Recently, Newburger and co-workers[15] found that a single 2 g/kg dose of IVIG showed a faster decrease in fever and laboratory parameters than a fractionated dose $(0.4 \, \mathrm{g \, kg^{-1} \, day^{-1}}$ on 4 consecutive days). Although the rapid reversal of the immunoregulatory abnormalities is almost coincident with resolution of fever and indices of inflammation[16], the anti-inflammatory effect seems to precede, as it is already apparent within the first day after IVIG[17], with the reduction of fever, white cell counts and levels of proteins associated with the acute phase. Pepsin-digested γ-globulin seems to be ineffective[13]. By day 4 the patients had a significant rise in Leu 2+ T cells ($p < 0.01$), a decrease

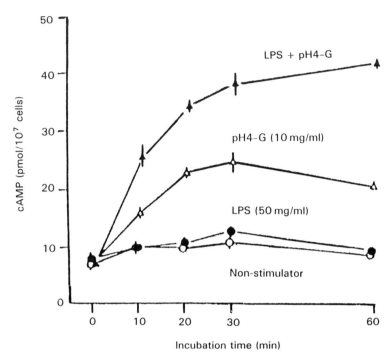

Figure 1 A possible mechanism of anti-inflammatory effect of intravenous immunoglobulin. Levels of intracellular cyclic adenosine monophosphate (cAMP) of peritoneal exudate cells (PEC) stimulated with lipopolysaccharide (LPS) and/or intravenous immunoglobulin, pH 4 (pH 4-G). Rabbit PEC (1×10^7) were incubated with or without LPS in the presence or absence of pH 4-G in a total volume of 0.5 ml for the time indicated. The amount of cAMP in the sample was measured by radioimmunoassay. Data are means ± SEM of the amount of cAMP in triplicate. Reproduced with permission from Shimozatu, T. *et al.* (1991). *Immunology*, **72**, 497-501

in Leu 3+ DR+ activated helper T cells ($p < 0.001$) and a decrease in spontaneous IgG secretion by circulating B lymphocytes ($p < 0.001$). Newburger and colleagues[18] suggest the possibility of a blockade of the immunological activation of the inflammatory response directed to vascular surfaces, and also consider a saturation of Fc receptors on platelets or reticuloendothelial cells, and do not discount the provision of a specific antibody to neutralize an unidentified etiological agent.

Behçet's disease is a complex vasculitis which may cause severe systemic symptoms. An enhanced neutrophil function or leukocytoclastic effect is characteristic. According to the 'tantalizing glimpses of some etiological factors'[19,20], Behçet's disease may be an autoimmune reaction triggered by viral, bacterial or other antigens. It is often responsive to immunosuppressive drugs, such as corticosteroids, chlorambucil, azathioprine and cyclosporin A. Interestingly, three cases of transient Behçet's disease were reported among neonates born to mothers with the disease[21]. Pregnancy in humans affords a valuable model for investigating the etiology and pathogenesis of autoimmune disease[22]. Women suffering from immunological diseases might be expected to transmit transitorily symptoms of the disease to their offspring, with two provisos:

(a) The IgG type antibody must make a significant contribution to the pathophysiology of the disease; and

(b) The fetal tissue must carry receptors for the antibody concerned.

This has been observed in autoimmune thrombocytopenia, Rh immunization and Graves' disease, and it occurs in about 12% of the infants born to myasthenic mothers[22]. In these conditions high-dose IVIG has been reported to be of benefit, and the only patient with Behçet's disease we had occasion to follow was treated apparently successfully. Aspirin was added to inhibit the platelet aggregator thromboxane, in order to counteract the increased potential for aggregation, to which the decreased prostacyclin sensitivity of platelets seems to contribute in patients with Behçet's syndrome[23].

Myasthenia gravis is a disorder characterized by fluctuating weakness and fatigue, and is provoked by a deficiency of acetylcholine receptor (AChR) at the neuromuscular junction. The clinical manifestations depend on the muscles involved and the disease severity. This tends to be most intense within the first 3 years from the onset of symptoms, followed by gradual improvement or, less often, a steady state. AChR antibodies are present in 85–90% of patients with myasthenia gravis[24]. The pathogenicity of AChR antibodies has been demonstrated most convincingly in passive transfer experiments. As mentioned previously, a mother with myasthenia gravis might transmit symptoms transitorily to her offspring. In addition, myasthenic antibodies may also activate complement, resulting in increased AChR destruction[25]. As in other autoimmune diseases, therapeutic strategies focus on the abnormal immune response and results are frequently satisfactory. Thymectomy is a specific option for this disease, with benefit for the majority of patients. High-dose IVIG, which has a distinct side-effect profile, has been proved to be a useful tool in the management of severe myasthenia gravis. Arsura[24] observed an improvement in 11 of 12 patients, beginning 3.6 ± 2.7 days after the start of the conventional dose of 0.4 g/kg on 5 consecutive days, becoming maximal in 8.4 ± 4.6 days, and lasting 52 ± 37 days. One patient became weaker, requiring endotracheal intubation and mechanical ventilation. The AChR antibody titer, which was elevated in all patients, remained unchanged after IVIG infusion and when sampled again after a month. The rapidity with which IVIG seems to act is equalled only by plasmapheresis, the difference being that in the latter the AChR antibody titer drops significantly. Kamolvarin and colleagues[25] observed that clinical improvement paralleled a decrement in C3c levels, suggesting that regulation of complement activation may be one possible mechanism of IVIG treatment in myasthenia gravis.

SLE is a prototype of an immune complex disease where immune complexes have been demonstrated in target tissues. Tomino and co-workers[26] demonstrated that glomerular immune complex deposits could be solubilized with human IgG. Palla and colleagues[27] treated four patients with membranous nephritis with IVIG, and had dramatic resolution of proteinuria in three of them. Reversible rises in serum creatinine have occasionally been seen after IVIG infusions in patients with nephrotic syndrome: however, IVIG has also been shown to reduce proteinuria in membranous nephropathy[28]. As already mentioned, Jordan[12] experienced an accentuation of glomerulonephritis with IVIG therapy in two SLE patients. Gaedicke and associates[29] reported an improvement in two acute vasculitic exacerbations in a patient treated with IVIG (we have had a similar experience), while in another, in whom arthralgia and morning stiffness prevailed, this therapy failed. At present we are following a 60-year-old female with SLE expressed mainly as generalized arthralgias and acceleration of erythrocyte sedimentation rate, who responds apparently well to prolonged therapy with high-dose IVIG, the symptoms exacerbating each time IVIG is interrupted for more than a month. In SLE-associated thrombocytopenia, Bussel and Hillgartner[30] refer to good results, whereas Cohen and Li[31] have found a prolonged, clinically worthwhile response in only two of 13 patients. Recently, Tomer and Shoenfeld[32] reported success with high-dose IVIG in the treatment of psychosis secondary to SLE. We may conclude that in this protean disease IVIG therapy is especially controversial. The reported cases with improvements suggest that its indication and dose adjustment have still to be determined.

The abating and painful 'idiopathic' inflammatory bowel diseases, which comprise ulcerative colitis and Crohn's disease, have a chronic evolution in which remissions and exacerbations are not rare. The etiology is unknown. It has been hypothesized that the immune system reacts inappropriately against a common antigen, possibly from the intestinal lumen. The pathology of the lesions, which includes infiltration of inflammatory cells, lymph-node hyperplasia and granulomas, plus the responsiveness to immunosuppressive drugs, and also the relatively frequent occurrence of circulating immune complexes, arthritis and uveitis, seems to validate the suspicion. Nevertheless, the possibility of an as yet undiscovered pathogen cannot be excluded. Ochs and colleagues[33] consider that the rationale for using IVIG is acceptable for both possibilities. Although the variable clinical course hampers the acceptance of case reports, high-dose IVIG therapy seems to spare corticosteroid requirements in some patients[33,34]. The anti-inflammatory effect of IVIG appears to be accountable, at least partially, for the improvement seen in patients with inflammatory bowel disease, as increased IL-1 production by activated intestinal lamina propria mononuclear cells has been found, and other lymphokines are supposed to be produced in excess locally. However, IVIG does not affect the root cause of the inflammation, and so the symptoms may return when it is withdrawn.

Among the diseases of the endocrine system we may include thyroid ophthalmopathy, which is often associated with Graves' hyperthyroidism, but which also occassionally occurs in patients with hypothyroidism, and even in those with Hashimoto's thyroiditis or in the absence of thyroid disease. When proptosis is severe, permanent damage to vision and ocular movement can result. The pathogenesis of thyroid eye disease is likely to be an autoimmune disease, although it has been demonstrated that thyroid-stimulating immunoglobulins and antibodies to thyroid-stimulating hormone receptors are not directly responsible. These patients are usually treated with large doses of corticosteroids, often with good results, although side-effects cannot be ignored. Irradiation of the orbit may give a transient or even prolonged relief, but carries the risk of cataract formation. High-dose IVIG offers an alternative. According to Dwyer and co-workers[35], at present it is the logical therapy of choice. They reported eight patients with advanced disease who experienced a subjective and objective clinical improvement. Also, Antonelli and colleagues[36] recently published that, in Graves' exophthalmos, the degree of ocular involvement

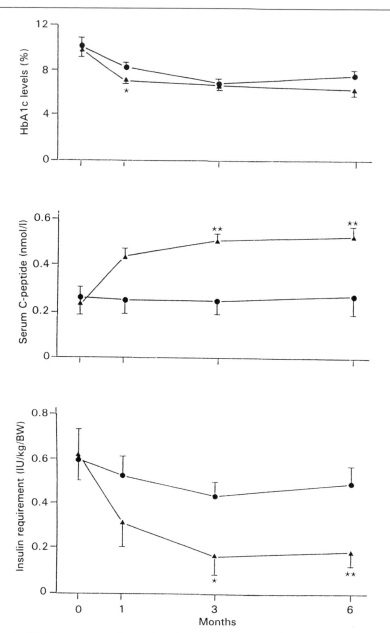

Figure 2 HbA1c percentage levels, insulin requirement (IU/kg/bw) and serum C-peptide levels (nmol/l) in control (●) and Ig-treated type 1 diabetic patients (▲). Values are mean ± SE. Significant differences are indicated; * p < 0.02; ** p < 0.01. Reproduced with permission from reference 37

response to IVIG showed a similar significant improvement, as with the X-ray treated group. Of course, these treatments will fail once the inflammatory process has declined and fibrotic changes become irreversible.

An attractive subject is juvenile type 1 diabetes mellitus, which has been demonstrated to be an autoimmune disorder. The functional efficiency of T-suppressor cells may be restored through IVIG. Previously, such findings were shown with cyclosporin A treatment. In newly diagnosed cases, Panto and associates[37] observed a reduction of insulin requirement in the 3rd ($p<0.02$) and even more so in the 6th month of IVIG therapy ($p < 0.005$). Of eight patients, two had a prolonged restoration of β-cell function, and insulin administration ceased. Serum C-peptide values were also significantly higher in the IVIG-treated group (Figure 2). Another observation was that islet-cell antibodies decreased in the IVIG-treated group, but not significantly compared with the control group. It is known that islet-cell antibodies may fluctuate during the first year of disease, and even disappear and reappear with low titers. The insulin-saving response was rather delayed. Less favorable are the results of Leong and colleagues[38], who showed a non-significant slowing in the fall of C-peptide responses to a glucagon meal test at 12 months and 24 months, but none of their patients who were followed for long enough had a clinical remission. Remarkably, they report that 80% of the infusions caused side-effects such as headache, nausea, lethargy, pyrexia and vomiting, and in 30% medical attention was sought. One may conclude that IVIG as treatment for insulin-dependent diabetes is still experimental.

After highlighting examples of the IVIG experience in autoimmune disease, I conclude that IVIG may be viewed as an active immunotherapy aimed at stimulating regulatory mechanisms which may herald a return to 'immune homeostasis', providing non-immunosuppressive approaches to the handling of autoimmune diseases. It may mimic the regulatory mechanism leading to a transitory or, occasionally, to a persistent down-regulation of pathological autoimmunity. In order to obtain a sustained benefit, it may be necessary to provide IVIG over a prolonged period of time, or permanently, at least until the underlying disease has been controlled or has remitted spontaneously. The difficulty lies in adjusting the dose to the individual disease process, hence the perils of over-simplification. An exacerbation of symptoms cannot be excluded, in spite of the apparent benefit in patients supposedly similar.

Bearing in mind the suffering of patients, it is my feeling that even anecdotal success cases are welcome, in spite of the failure rate and the fact that spontaneous remissions may occur.

REFERENCES

1. Sultan, Y., Kazatchkine, M. D., Maisonneuve, P. and Nydegger, U. E. (1984). Anti-idiotypic suppression of autoantibodies to factor VIII (anti-haemophilic factor) by high-dose intravenous γ-globulin. *Lancet*, **2**, 765–8
2. Heyman, M. R., Chakravarthy, A., Edelman, B. B. *et al.* (1988). Failure of high-dose i.v. γ-globulin in the treatment of spontaneously acquired factor VIII inhibitors. *Am. J. Hematol.*, **28**, 191–4
3. Rossi, F., Sultan, Y. and Kazatchkine, M. D. (1988). Anti-idiotypes against autoantibodies and alloantibodies to VIII:C (anti-haemophilic factor) are present in therapeutic polyspecific normal immunoglobulins. *Clin. Exp. Immunol.*, **74**, 311–16
4. Nilson, M., Sundquist, S. B., Ljung, R. *et al.* (1983). Suppression of secondary antibody response by intravenous immunoglobulin in patients with haemophilia B and antibodies. *Scand. J. Haematol.*, **30**, 458–64
5. Moffat, E. H., Furlong, R. A., Dannatt, A. H. G. *et al.* (1989). Anti-idiotypes to factor VIII antibodies and their possible role in the pathogenesis and treatment of factor VIII inhibitors. *Br. J. Haematol.*, **71**, 85–90
6. Rewald, E. (1992). Intravenous immunoglobulin and spontaneous hemorrhage in a case of Factor VIII inhibitor. Presented at the *24th Congress of the International Society of Haematology*, London, UK, August 1992, Abstract 1596
7. Annetta, I., Otaso, J., Nucifora, E. *et al.* (1992). Inhibidor de factor VIII postparto: presentatión de 2 casos. *4a Reunión Científica 1992, Soc. Arg. Hematology*
8. Macik, B. G., Gabriel, D. A., White, G. C., High, K. and Roberts, H. (1988). The use of high-dose intravenous γ-globulin in acquired von Willebrand syndrome. *Arch. Pathol. Lab. Med.*, **112**, 143–6
9. Wong, P., Itoh, K. and Yoshida, S. (1986). Treatment of thrombotic thrombocytopenic purpura with intravenous γ-globulin. *N. Engl. J. Med.*, **314**, 385–6
10. Stricker, R. B. and Kiprov, D. D. (1991). Combined use of plasmapheresis and intravenous γ-globulin in the treatment of HIV-positive and HIV-negative autoimmune syndromes. In Imbach, P. (ed.) *Immunotherapy with Intravenous Immunoglobulins*, pp. 345–9. (London:Academic Press)
11. Jayne, D. R. W., Davied, M. J., Fox, C. J. V. *et al.* (1991). Treatment of systemic vasculitis with pooled intravenous immunoglobulin. *Lancet*, **337**, 1137–9

12. Jordan, S. C. (1989). Intravenous γ-globulin therapy in systemic lupus erythematosus and immune complex disease. *Clin. Immunol. Immunopathol.*, **53**, S164–S169

13. Shulman, S. T. (1991). Kawasaki disease and IVIG: what's going on here? In Imbach, P. (ed.) *Immunotherapy with Intravenous Immunoglobulins*, pp. 261–8. (London:Academic Press)

14. Furusho K., Kamiya, T., Nakano, H. *et al.* (1984). High-dose intravenous γ-globulin for Kawasaki disease. *Lancet*, **2**, 1055–8

15. Newburger, J. W. and US Multicenter Kawasaki Study Group. (1990). Preliminary results of multicenter trial of IVIG treatment of Kawasaki disease with single infusion vs. four-infusion regimen. *Pediatr. Res.*, **27**, 22A (Abstract no 119)

16. Leung, D. Y. M., Burns, J. C., Newbeuger, J. W. *et al.* (1987). Reversal from lymphocyte activation *in vivo* in the Kawasaki syndrome by intravenous γ-globulin. *J. Clin. Invest.*, **79**, 468–72

17. Eibl, M. M. (1990). γ-Globulin therapy. *Curr. Opin. Pediatr.*, 935–40

18. Newburger, J. W., Takahashi, M., Burns, J. C. *et al.* (1986). The treatment of Kawasaki syndrome with intravenous γ-globulin. *N. Engl. J. Med.*, **315**, 341–7

19. Cobby, M., Higgs, C. M. B. and Hall, C. L. (1988). Behçet's syndrome presenting as intracranial hypertension in a Caucasian. *J. Roy. Soc. Med.*, **81**, 478–9

20. Editorial. (1989). Behçet's disease. *Lancet*, **1**, 761–2

21. Lewis, M. A. and Priestley, B. L. (1986). Transient neonatal Behçet's disease. *Arch. Dis. Child.*, **61**, 805–6

22. Head, J. R. and Billingham, R. E. (1982). Immunobiological aspects of maternal-fetoplacental relationship. In Lachmann, P. J. and Peters, D. K. (eds.) *Clinical Aspects of Immunology*, pp. 243–82. (Oxford:Blackwell Scientific)

23. Rewald, E. and Jakcic, J. C. (1990). Behçet's syndrome treated with high-dose intravenous IgG and low-dose aspirin. *J. Roy. Soc. Med.*, **83**, 652–3

24. Arsura, E. (1989). Experience with intravenous immunoglobulin in myasthenia gravis. *Clin. Immunol. Immunopathol.*, **53**, 170–9

25. Kamolvarin, N., Hemachudha, T., Ongpipattanakul, B. *et al.* (1989). Plasma C3c changes in myasthenia gravis patients receiving high-dose intravenous immunoglobulin during crisis. *Acta Neurol. Scand.*, **80**, 324–6

26. Tomino, Y., Sakai, H., Takaya, M. *et al.* (1984). Solubilization of intraglomerular deposits of IgG immune complexes by human sera or γ-globulin in patients with lupus nephritis. *Clin. Exp. Immunol.*, **58**, 42–8

27. Palla, R., Cirami, C., Panichi, V. *et al.* (1991). Intravenous immunoglobulin therapy of membranous nephropathy: efficacy and safety. *Clin. Nephrol.*, **35**, 98–104

28. Schifferli, J. A. (1992). High-dose intravenous immunoglobulin treatment and renal function. In Dominioni, L. and Nydegger, U. E. (eds.) *Intravenous Immunoglobulins Today and Tomorrow*, pp. 27–33. (London:Royal Society of Medicine Services Ltd.)

29. Gaedicke, G., Teller, W. M., Kohne, E. *et al.* (1984). IgG therapy in systemic lupus erythematosus. *Blut*, **48**, 387–90

30. Bussel, J. B. and Hillgartner, M. W. (1987). Intravenous immunoglobulin therapy of idiopathic thrombocytopenic purpura in childhood and adolescence. *Hematol. Oncol. Clin. N. Am.*, **1**, 465–82

31. Cohen, M. G. and Li, E. K. (1991). Limited effects of intravenous IgG in treating systemic lupus erythematosus-associated thrombocytopenia. *Arthritis Rheumatism*, **34**, 787–8

32. Tomer, Y. and Shoenfeld, Y. (1992). Successful treatment of psychosis secondary to SLE with high dose intravenous immunoglobulin. *Clin. Exp. Rheumatol.*, **10**, 391–4

33. Ochs, H., Fischer, S. H., Christie, D. L. *et al.* (1991). Intravenous immunoglobulin in idiopathic inflammatory bowel disease: results of an open-label therapeutic trial. In Imbach, P. (ed.) *Immunotherapy with Intravenous Immunoglobulins*, pp. 359–76. (London:Academic Press)

34. Knoflach, P., Müller, C. and Eibl, M. M. (1990). Crohn disease and intravenous immunoglobulin G. *Ann. Intern. Med.*, **112**, 385–6

35. Dwyer, J. M., Benson, E. M., Currie, J. N. *et al.* (1991). Intravenously administered IgG for the treatment of thyroid eye disease. In Imbach P. (ed.) *Immunotherapy with Intravenous Immunoglobulins*, pp. 387–94. (London: Academic Press)

36. Antonelli, A., Saracino, A., Alberti, B. *et al.* (1992). High-dose intravenous immunoglobulin treatment in Graves' ophthalmopathy. *Acta Endocrinol.*, **126**, 13–23

37. Panto, F., Giordano, C., Amato, M. P. *et al.* (1990). The influence of high dose intravenous immunoglobulins on immunological and metabolic pattern in newly diagnosed type I diabetic patients. *J. Autoimmun.*, **3**, 587–92

38. Leong, G. M., Thayer, Z., Antony, G. *et al.* (1991). High-dose intravenous immunoglobulin therapy for insulin-dependent diabetes mellitus. In Imbach, P. (ed.) *Immunotherapy with Intravenous Immunoglobulins*, pp. 269–82. (London:Academic Press)

19

Current developments in the treatment of autoimmune diseases

H. Borberg, C. Jimenez, W. F. Haupt and F. Rosenow

The standard therapy of autoimmune diseases consists of immuno-suppressive drugs, mainly corticosteroids and cytostatics such as azathioprine, methotrexate or cyclophosphamide. However, their application is limited, due to dose-dependent side-effects such as Cushing's syndrome, myelosuppression, cystitis, liver fibrosis etc. Alternative therapies are therefore highly desirable. At present, extracorporeal elimination therapy, immunomodulation and a combination of both are available.

Extracorporeal elimination is generally performed by separating plasma from cells by centrifugation with blood (cell) separators, or by filtration using sheet membranes or hollow fibers. We prefer centrifugation, for a number of reasons:

(1) Continuous or discontinuous centrifugation is generally performed from one antecubital vein to the other, avoiding artificial access to the circulation such as a shunt or Shaldon catheter, thereby excluding dangerous access-related side-effects.

(2) The separation is more effective, as high g forces permit the concentration of cells to a hematocrit allowing for a plasma flow-rate between 20% and 30% higher than filtration procedures. If the appropriate centrifugation systems are applied, high g forces provide for virtually platelet-free plasma.

(3) As the disposable costs are generally less than 50% of those of filtration procedures, centrifugation is more economical.

Table 1 Established and debatable indications for plasma exchange therapy: immunological diseases

Antibody-mediated diseases
  Goodpasture's syndrome
  Hemophilia with antibody
  Autoimmune hemolytic anemia
  Idiopathic thrombocytopenia
  Rh–immunization
  Myasthenia gravis pseudoparalytica
  Pemphigus vulgaris
  Herpes gestationis
  Antibody-mediated transplant rejection (kidney, bone marrow)

Immune complex-mediated diseases
  Rapid progressive glomerulonephritis
  Hemophilia with immune complexes
  Dermatomyositis
  Scleroderma
  Immune vasculitis
    Lupus erythematosus disseminatus
    Panarteritis nodosa
    Allergic angiitis
    Wegener's granulomatosis

Unknown immune pathogenesis or highly debatable indications
  Morbus Raynaud
  Primary chronic polyarthritis
  Thrombotic thrombocytopenic purpura (Moschcowitz)
  Acute and chronic polyneuritis (Guillain–Barré)
  'Autoimmune' uveitis

Extracorporeal elimination therapy may be non-specific, selective or specific. We define a procedure as non-specific if the pathogenic substrate is eliminated with virtually all plasma proteins. A selective technique cannot be performed without losing some normal plasma proteins together with the pathogenic factor. The specific approach restricts the elimination exclusively to the undesired substrate.

Plasma exchange therapy is a typical example of non-specific elimination. An overview of the established and debatable indications is given in Table 1. Selective elimination techniques concentrating mainly on the elimination of immunoglobulins have recently been developed and improved[1-8]. These are based either on hydrophobic interaction chromatography or on affinity chromatography. The carrier material is either polyvinylalcohol, sepharose or silica. Ligands are amino acids such as tryptophan, phenylalanine, protein A or anti-Ig antibodies. The ligands are generally covalently coupled to the carrier material (Table 2). The adsorption columns applied differ in their volume, capacity and selectivity.

The selectivity is of special interest. It may be related to the capacity of the system, as the removal of normal plasma constituents such as fibrinogen may limit the efficacy of a single treatment. As illustrated in Table 3, hydrophobic interaction chromatography using Tryptophan 350 (TR 350) columns (Asahi Medical) is hampered badly by the loss of fibrinogen. This table also demonstrates that virtually all selective adsorbents remove all types of immunoglobulins (the TR 350 also eliminates IgE) and also albumin to a certain extent. If one looks at the IgG subfractions (Table 4), it is most interesting to observe that the different adsorbers behave quite differently. IgG2 and IgG4 are eliminated poorly from the tryptophan adsorber. In contrast, the protein-A columns[1] hardly eliminate IgG3. The anti-Ig adsorber eliminates all subclasses to the same extent. Whether this has any clinical relevance is not known so far; however, one may speculate that it could be meaningful for the treatment of immune complex-mediated diseases.

Table 5 summarizes the indications for selective adsorption. It is interesting that this overview is similar to that of plasma exchange. In our department, plasma exchange has indeed been widely replaced by selective adsorption therapy.

We know by experience that the extracorporeal treatment of auto-immune diseases does not suffice to control the course of the disease. As the extracorporeal approach removes only the produced substrate but does not down-regulate the substrate synthesis in the corresponding clone of cells, additional therapy attempting to suppress the pathogenic substrate production is needed. The limitations of drug-mediated immunosuppression have already been mentioned. In contrast, specific immunoregulation using monoclonal antibodies is hardly developed. So far, the most impressive results have been achieved with the introduction of intravenously applied 7 S immunoglobulins. Imbach's initial report in the *Lancet*[9] stimulated and still stimulates an impressive series

Table 2 Characteristics of selective plasma protein adsorption

	Adsorber			
	TR 350	PH 350	Protein A	Anti-IgG
Principle	hydrophobic interaction	hydrophobic interaction chromatography	affinity chromatography	affinity chromatography
Volume of column (ml)	350	350	62.5	400
Capacity (/l plasma)	2–2.5	2–2.5	(4)*	0.9–10**
Carrier material	polyvinyl alcohol	polyvinyl alcohol	sepharose silica	sepharose
Coupling of ligand	covalent	covalent	covalent	covalent

* Capacity of the system = repeated loading; ** = repeated loading possible

Table 3 Selective adsorption of plasma proteins: decrease with so-called immunoglobulin (Ig) adsorbers per liter of plasma (n = 10)

Adsorber	Albumin		Fibrinogen		IgG		IgM		IgA		Total protein	
	(g/l)	(%)	(mg/dl)	(%)	(g/l)	(%)	(g/l)	(%)	(g/l)	(%)	(g/l)	(%)
TR 350	4.25	11.2	133.3	49.7	2.73	31.4	0.43	30.2	0.51	19.0	2.73	31.4
Protein A	6.09	15.8	50.9	17.4	5.62	65.6	0.32	35.6	0.59	33.7	5.62	65.6
Anti-Ig	8.31	21.1	38.1	14.6	3.44	34.3	0.46	31.5	0.68	31.3	3.44	34.3

Table 4 Selective adsorption of plasma proteins: decrease of IgG subclasses in % per liter of plasma ($n = 10$)

Adsorber	IgG1	IgG2	IgG3	IgG4
TR 350	81.6	9.9	6.5	1.8
Protein A	63.2	29.5	0.7	6.6
Anti-Ig	67.0	20.6	5.9	6.4

Table 5 Indications for selective or specific plasma adsorption therapy

Immunological diseases
Antibody-mediated diseases
  Goodpasture's syndrome
  Myasthenia gravis pseudoparalytica
  Hemophilia with antibody
  Antibody-mediated transplant rejection
  ABO-incompatible bone marrow transplantation
Debatable pathogenesis
  Acute polyneuropathy Guillain–Barré

Exogenous intoxications
Digoxin apheresis

Metabolic diseases
Familial hypercholesterolemia (low–density lipoprotein immune apheresis)
Refsum's syndrome

of anecdotal reports, as well as controlled trials demonstrating the usefulness of this approach, in spite of the fact that the underlying mechanism has so far not been completely elucidated.

It appears that extracorporeal therapy and unspecific immunomodulation using 7 S immunoglobulins are competing approaches for the control of autoimmune diseases beyond immunosuppression by drugs. However, according to our observations, the sequential application of extracorporeal elimination plus subsequent intravenous immunoglobulin infusions is superior to either approach[10-12]. This is nicely demonstrated in both acute and chronic autoimmune thrombocytopenia, in which the efficacy of the treatment can be monitored by the platelet count.

Figure 1 shows all three types of response in the same patient suffering from refractory chronic autoimmune thrombocytopenia (AITP). An increase < 10 000 up to 38 000 platelets/μl follows selective adsorption. An increase beyond 50 000 can be observed after 30 g IgG (Sandoglobulin®, Sandoz) given intravenously over 5 days, and subsequently the response after three selective adsorptions followed by a 5-day infusion period of 30 g IgG/day is demonstrated.

Figure 2 shows the situation of a patient with chronic AITP treated with adsorption and 7 S immunoglobulin to permit both coronary angiography and by-pass operation. The high level of platelets beyond 300 000 caused the surgeon to treat him with pyridamole. This patient needed no further treatment for the next few months, was splenectomized, relapsed and is now under long-term observation. Whenever his platelet count falls below 20 000, he is successfully treated with a regular dose of immunoglobulin.

A summary of the treatment results in patients with acute auto-immune thrombocytopenic purpura is given in Table 6. Due to the small numbers of patients, however, no conclusion is possible but the two patients treated with the combined modality responded much better than the others. The superiority of the combined approach is demonstrated in Table 7, which compares this with extracorporeal therapy and immunoglobulin therapy separately.

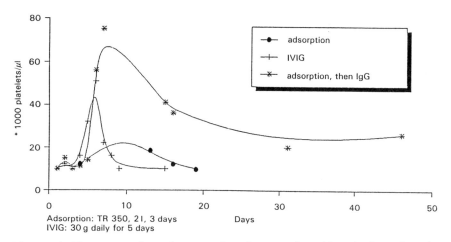

Figure 1 Treatment of autoimmune thrombocytopenia with selective adsorption, immunoglobulins and sequential combination of both. IVIG, intravenous immunoglobulin

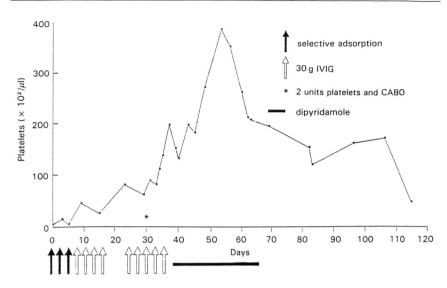

Figure 2 The clinical efficacy of combining selective tryptophan-mediated adsorption and 30 g intravenous immunoglobulin (IVIG) in a patient with autoimmune thrombocytopenia. CABO, coronary artery bypass operation

It was quite surprising that the combination of selective adsorption and Sandoglobulin® (Sandoz) was less effective than plasma exchange combined with 7 S IgG. In the search for an explanation we looked for the relation between clinical result and immunoglobulin depletion prior to immunoglobulin infusion, and found a correlation between both[4]. It is not yet clear whether this is a correlation between clinical effect and IgG with or without additional IgM depletion; however, due to this preliminary observation we changed our approach by depleting the IgG prior to infusion to the lowest possible value, and this in fact appears to provide for better data than just eliminating a pathogenic substrate on a volume per treatment basis, as is generally performed.

With this approach we have also treated a limited number of patients with immune complex-mediated diseases. So far, two patients with immune vasculitis, two with Wegener's disease and three with lupus erythematosus have been treated successfully, mainly with a combination of plasma exchange and subsequent Sandoglobulin® (Sandoz) infusion. In collaboration with the Department of Neurology of the University of Cologne, we have also treated patients with acute Guillain–Barré syndrome.

Table 6 Preliminary results of different treatment regimens in acute autoimmune thrombocytopenic purpura

| | Plasma exchange | | Selective adsorption (n = 1) | 7S IVIG (n = 3) | Plasma exchange + 7S IVIG (n = 0) | Selective adsorption + 7S IVIG (n = 2) |
	Albumin (n = 1)	Serum (n = 1)				
Average platelet count at hospitalization (10³/µl)	10	<10	10	<10	—	<10
Maximal platelet count after therapy (10³/µl)	21.5 (11–32)*	95	53	52 (41–63)*	—	160

* Range

Table 7 Results of different treatment regimens in chronic autoimmune thrombocytopenic purpura

| | Plasma exchange | | Selective adsorption (n = 6)* | 7S IVIG (n = 7) | Plasma exchange + 7S IVIG (n = 2) | Selective adsorption + 7S IVIG (n = 9) |
	Albumin (n = 1)	Serum (n = 4)				
Platelet count at hospitalization (10³/µl)	15	10	<10	<10	10	<10
Maximal platelet count after therapy (10³/µl)	27	21 (10–32)**	28 (12–60)	48 (32–60)	158 (136–180)	86 (11–140)

* Two patients treated with TR 350, two with protein A, two with anti-Ig columns; ** range

Table 8   Treatment trials in acute Guillain–Barré syndrome

Steroids
Stillman *et al.* (1952)
Swick *et al.* (1976)
Hughes *et al.* (1978)[14]
Hughes (1991)[15]

Immunoglobulins
Kleyweg *et al.* (1988)
Van der Meché *et al.* (1992)[18]

Plasma exchange
Guillain–Barré Study Group (1985)[13]
French Cooperative Group (1987)

Immunoadsorption
Pencz and Garnier (1990)[17]

Table 8 summarizes the different trials for the treatment of acute Guillain–Barré syndrome, representing the present state of the art. As steroids have not shown to be at all successful, plasma exchange and the intravenous application of immunoglobulins are the therapies of choice at the present time[13-17]. So far, no precise information on the superiority of either treatment is available. An attempt to replace plasma exchange therapy by selective adsorption was described by Pencz and Garnier in 1990[17], without answering the question whether this was superior or inferior.

Based on our earlier experience in treating myasthenia gravis with selective adsorption rather than plasma exchange therapy[2,3,19] we also treated patients with acute Guillain–Barré syndrome with hydrophobic interaction chromatography using the Asahi TR 350 adsorber. In a retrospective study, three groups of patients were compared with each other. One group received a symptomatic treatment only, another group was treated with plasma exchange and a third group was treated with selective adsorption using the Asahi TR 350 adsorber. As can be seen from Table 9, all groups were fairly homogeneous. Table 9 clearly demonstrates the superiority of the extracorporeal therapy, compared to the symptomatic treatment. Statistical evaluation using the Kruskal–Wallis and the Freeman–Halton tests shows the corresponding statistical

Table 9 Clinical course of 37 acute matched Guillain–Barré syndrome patients with different treatments. Average time in days

Treatment group only	Plasma exchange (n = 11)	Adsorption (TR 350) (n = 7)	Adsorption + IVIG (n = 9)	Symptomatic treatment (n = 10)	
From onset to 1st improvement	16.7	14.7	21.3	20.1	NS
Time in hospital	82.2	49.8	64.3	98.5	NS
Interval from 1st treatment to 1st improvement	5.3	3.6	7.5	0	
Disability score on discharge	1.3	1.1	1.2	1.0	NS

NS, not significant

Table 10 Procedural complications in 27 acute Guillian–Barré syndrome patients with different plasma treatments (n = 10 for each treatment group)

Side-effects	Plasma exchange	Adsorption (TR 350)	Adsorption + IgG
Fibrinogen < 50 mg%	2	1	0
PTT and/or PT > 2 min	2	2	0
Fall in blood pressure > 40 mmHg	4	2	1
Rise in blood pressure > 40 mmHg	2	0	0
Chills, urticaria, paresthesiae	6	2	1
Angina pectoris	0	1	0
Others (possibly related)	0	1*	0

* Stroke 2 h after therapy; PTT, partial thromboplastin time; PT, prothrombin time

significances (Table 10). There was no difference in side-effects between groups. We thus conclude that selective adsorption is capable of replacing plasma exchange therapy. However, the question as to whether immunoglobulins may play an additional role also needs to be answered.

Table 9 demonstrates that the combined approach is also competitive to plasma exchange and adsorption therapy.

In conclusion, it is obvious that extracorporeal elimination and IVIG are superior to symptomatic therapy. Our anecdotal data do not demonstrate the superiority of the extracorporeal treatment approaches against each other. However, they also do not lead to deterioration. Selective adsorption appears to be equal to plasma exchange and IVIG therapy seems to compete with extracorporeal elimination therapy. If both extracorporeal elimination and immunomodulation with 7 S immunoglobulins are effective therapies, a sequential application appears to be reasonable, and we therefore suggest a controlled trial comparing adsorption with immunomodulation with the combined approach. To make this trial possible, an improved system of clinical assessment has been developed[12,20].

We were rather disappointed that the retrospective analysis did not demonstrate a clear superiority of the combined approach compared to either immunoglobulin therapy or extracorporeal elimination. Trying to correlate the clinical results with the extent of the extracorporeal therapy, we found again that there appears to be a relation between the extent of IgG and/or IgM depletion and clinical outcome[4]. We are currently engaged in a retrospective analysis of this correlation, and also prospectively, using IgG depletion as a predictive parameter rather than working on a volume-based approach.

As the last three patients not yet included in Table 9, treated with a more aggressive and predictable lowering of IgG and IgM followed by the standard immunoglobulin therapy, left the hospital after 2 weeks, we feel that such lowered IgG and/or IgM titers may well lead to a further improvement of the clinical results, and that the correlation with the elimination of immunoglobulins permits a better prediction of results.

Whereas acute Guillain–Barré syndrome appears to improve rapidly, little progress is observed in the treatment of chronic inflammatory demyelinating polyneuropathy (CIDP). The problems in the assessment of the treatment are the small number of patients, the unknown

Table 11 Chronic inflammatory demyelinating polyneuropathy: treatment results with hemapheresis

Reference	No. of patients	No. of relapses	No. of treatments	Treatment effect	Other medications
Server et al.[22]	1	3	3 + 4 + 2	1 +	steroids
Levy et al.[23]	1	1	4	1 +	steroids, ACTH
Dalakas et al.[24]	3	1	4	1 + , 2 −	steroids
Gross et al.[25]	2		4, 7	1 + , 1 −	steroids
Gross et al.[26]	6	3 relapses 3 progressions		3 + 3 −	steroids, cyclophosphamide, azathioprine, cyclosporin
Dyck et al.	7		6	4 + , 3 −	
Dyck et al.[21]	15			8 +	comparison with 8 sham PE
Pollard et al.[27]	5		8–20 (1 cont.)	2 + , 3 −	steroids, azathioprine, cyclophosphamide
Feasby et al.[28]	5		cont.	5 +	
Gibbels et al.[29]	9	7 relapses 2 progressions	12	4 + , 3 − 2 −	steroids, azathioprine, cyclophosphamide
Bönner et al.[30]	2	multiple	6, 8	1 + , 1 −	steroids, azathioprine
Maas et al.[31]	1	multiple	3	1 +	steroids, azathioprine
Cook et al.[32]	3	>2	5	3 +	steroids, azathioprine
Total	60			35 + /25 −	

ACTH, adrenocorticotropic hormone; PE, plasma exchange

214

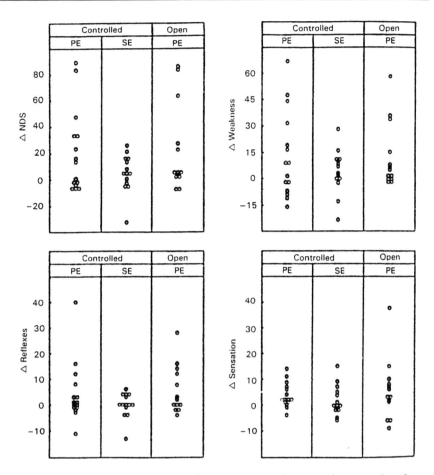

Figure 3 Treatment results in chronic inflammatory demyelinating polyneuropathy: plasma exchange vs. sham exchange. Changes in neurological disability score (NDS) and in the tendon reflexes, weakness, and sensation subsets of the neurological disability score 3 weeks after plasma exchange (PE) or sham exchange (SE) in the controlled trial and after plasma exchange in the open trial. Each symbol represents the response of one patient. Positive values indicate improvement. Reproduced with permission from Dyck *et al.*[21]

pathogenesis, the multiple subtypes of the disease, the lack of predictors, the difficult clinical grading and the variability of the treatment regimens. A review of the literature (Table 11) hints at some advantage of plasma exchange (Figure 3) therapy, as does a trial of plasma exchange versus sham exchange published by Dyck in 1986[21]. This correlates with our own experience; however, it must be stated clearly that all these data do not suffice to give a recommendation for any particular treatment modality. We have treated one patient with IVIG during a relapse of the disease and found a quite positive response, leading to speculation that CIDP may also respond to immunoglobulins, and that a sequential approach might be even more useful.

We have also recently begun to treat patients with myasthenia gravis in combination with subsequent immunoglobulin therapy. Two patients treated so far have responded; however, since the number of patients has decreased drastically following the introduction of extracorporeal elimination therapy, it will be difficult to obtain a sufficiently clear response during the next couple of years.

REFERENCES

1. Bansal, S. C., Bansal, B. R., Thomas, H. L., Siegal, P. D., Rhoads, J. E. Jr., Cooper, D. R., Terman, D. S. and Mark, R. (1978). *Ex vivo* removal of serum IgG in a patient with colon carcinoma. *Cancer*, **42**, 1–18
2. Heininger, K., Toyka, K.V., Gaczkowski, A., Hartung, H. P. and Borberg, H. (1987). Therapeutic plasma exchange in myasthenia gravis: semi-selection adsorption of anti-AChR autoantibodies with tryptophan-linked polyvinylalcohol gels. *Ann. N.Y. Acad. Sci.*, 898–900
3. Heininger, K., Toyka, K. V., Gaczkowski, A., Hartung, H. P., Borberg, H. and Grabensee, B. (1986). Selective removal of pathogenic factors in neurological diseases. *Plasma Ther. Transfus. Technol.*, **7**, 351–7
4. Jiménez-Klingberg, C., Rosenow, F., Grieb, P., Haupt, W. F. and Borberg, H. (1991). Adsorption therapy with trytophan conjuated polyvinyl alcohol gels in 10 patients with acute Guillain–Barré syndrome. *Infusionstherapie*, **18** (Suppl. 2), 44
5. Jiménez-Klingberg, C. (1992). Selection adsorption of immunoglobulin G: a comparison of a new type of adsorber with protein A and trytophan conjugated polyvinylalcohol gel columns. *4th International Congress of the World Apheresis Association*, Sapporo, June 3–5
6. Nilsson, I. M., Johnson, S., Sundquist, S. B., Ahlberg, A. and Bergentz, S. E. (1981). A procedure for removing high titer antibodies by extracorporeal protein-A-sepharose adsorption in hemophilia: substitution therapy and surgery in a patient with hemophilia B and antibodies. *Blood*, **38**, 44
7. Ray, P. K., Idiculla, A., Rhoads, J. E. Jr., Besa E., Bassett, J. C. and Cooper, D. R. (1980). Immunoadsorption of IgG molecules from the plasma of

multiple myeloma and autoimmune hemolytic anemia patients. *Plasma Ther.*, **1**, 11–17

8. Rosenow, F., Haupt, W. F., Neveling, M., Grieb, P., Jiménez, C. and Borberg, H. (1991). Plasma exchange and selective adsorption in Guillain–Barré syndrome. A comparison of therapy by clinical course and side effects. *Infusionstherapie*, **18** (Suppl. 2), 45

9. Imbach, P., Barandum, S., d'Appuzo, V., Baumgartner, C., Hirt, A., Morell, A., Rossi, E., Schöni, M., Vest, M. and Wagner, H. P. (1981). High-dose intravenous γ-globulin for idiopathic thrombocytopenic purpura in childhood. *Lancet*, **1**, 1228–31

10. Borberg, H., Gaczkowski, A., Kadar, J. and Brunner, G. (1990). Immunomodulatory extracorporal elimination therapy for the treatment of autoimmune diseases. *Third International Congress of the World Apheresis Association*, Amsterdam, April 9–12. Abstract

11. Borberg, H. (1993). Die extrakorporale Eliminationsbehandlung von Autoimmunerkrankungen. *Workshop on Haemofiltration, Haemodialysis and Haemapheresis*, Salzberg, May 13–15, in press

12. Haupt, W. F., Borberg, H. and Rosenow, F. (1992). A new treatment concept for acute Guillain–Barré syndrome: basis for a multicenter study. *J. Neurol.*, **239** (Suppl. 3), 46

13. Guillain–Barré syndrome Study Group. (1985). Plasmapheresis and acute Guillain–Barré syndrome. *Neurology*, **35**, 1096–104

14. Hughes R. A. C., Newson-Davis J. M., Perkin G. D. and Pierce J. M. (1978). Controlled trial of prednisolone in acute polyneuropathy. *Lancet*, **2**, 750–3

15. Hughes, R. A. C. (1991). Ineffectiveness of high-dose intravenous methyl-prednisolone in Guillain–Barré syndrome. *Lancet*, **338**, 1142

16. NIH Consensus Conference. (1990). Intravenous immunoglobulin: prevention and treatment of disease. *J. Am. Med. Assoc.*, **264**, 3189–93

17. Pencz, A. and Garnier, A. (1990). Immunadsorption in der Behandlung der Polyradikulitis vom Typ Guillain–Barré. *Nervenarzt*, **61**, 372–5

18. Van der Meché, F. G. A., Schmitz, P. I. M. and the Dutch Guillain–Barré Study Group. (1992). A randomized trial comparing intravenous immune globulin and plasma exchange in Guillain–Barré syndrome. *N. Engl. J. Med.*, **326**, 1123–9

19. Sato, T., Nishimiya, J., Arai, K., Anno, M., Yamawaki, N., Kuroda, T. and Inagaki, K. (1983). Selective removal of anti-acetylcholine receptor antibodies in sera from patients with myasthenia gravis *in vitro* with a new immunoadsorbent. In Oda, T. (ed.) *3rd Symposium on Therapeutic Plasmapheresis, Tokyo. Therapeutic Plasmapheresis (III)*, pp. 565–8. (Stuttgart: Schattauer Verlag)

20. Rosenow, F., Haupt, W. F., Rose, A. and Borberg, H. (1992). The paresis score – a new instrument for the prospective documentation of the clinical course in 30 patients with Guillain–Barré syndrome and CIDP. *J. Neurol.*, **239** (Suppl. 3), 49

21. Dyck, P. J., Daube, J., O'Brien, P., Pineda, A., Low, P. A., Windebaute, A. J. and Swanson, C. (1986). Plasma exchange in chronic inflammatory demyelinating polyradiculoneuropathy. *N. Engl. J. Med.*, **314**, 461–5

22. Server, A. C., Lefkowith, J., Braine, H. and McKhann, G. M., (1979). Treatment of chronic relapsing inflammatory polyradiculoneuropathy by plasma exchange. *Ann. Neurol.*, **6**, 258–61

23. Levy, R., Newkirk, R. and Ochoa, J. (1979). Treatment of chronic relapsing Guillain–Barré syndrome by plasma exchange. *Lancet*, **2**, 741

24. Dalakas, J. D., McLeod, J. G., Gatenby, P. and Kronenberg, H., (1981). Polyneuropathy: pathogenesis and therapy *Ann. Neurol*, **9** (Suppl.), 134–45

25. Gross, M. L. P., Legg, N. J., Lockwood, M. C. and Pallis, C. (1982). The treatment of inflammatory polyneuropathy by plasma exchange. *J. Neurol. Neurosurg. Psychiatr.*, **45**, 675–9

26. Gross, M. L. P. and Thomas, P. K. (1981). The treatment of chronic relapsing and chronic progressive idiopathic inflammatory polyneuropathy by plasma exchange. *J. Neurol. Sci.*, **52**, 69–78

27. Pollard, J. D., McLeod, J. G., Gatenby, P. and Kronenberg, H. (1983). Prediction of response to plasma exchange in chronic relapsing polyneuropathy. *J. Neurol. Sci.*, **58**, 269–87

28. Feasby, T. E., Halm, A. F. and Brown, W. F. (1983). Long-term plasmapheresis in chronic progressive demyelinating polyneuropathy. *Ann. Neurol.*, **14**, 122

29. Gibbels, E., Toyka, K. V., Borberg, H., Hapt, W. F. and Hann, P. (1986). Plasmaaustauschbehandlung bei chronischen Polyneuritiden vom Typ Guillain–Barré. *Nervenarzt*, **57**, 129–39

30. Bönner, G., Bewermeyer, H., Aboudan, F., Renner, E., Heiss, W. D. and Kaufmann, W. (1984). Plasmapheresetherapie der akuten und chronischen Polyradikuloneuritis. *Therapiewoche*, **34**, 153–8

31. Maas, A. I. R., Busch, H. F. M. and van de Heul, C. (1981). Plasma infusion and plasma exchange in chronic idiopathic polyneuropathy. *N. Engl. J. Med.*, **30**, 344

32. Cook, J. D., Tindall R. A. S., Walker, J., Khan, A. and Rosenberg, R. (1980). Plasma exchange as a treatment of acute and chronic idiopathic autoimmune polyneuropathy: limited success. *Neurology*, **30**, 361

20

Intravenous immunoglobulin and autoimmunity

J. M. Dwyer

INTRODUCTON

Evolutionary pressures from the potentially hostile world of micro-organisms have resulted in the development of a sophisticated defensive repertoire (immune system) capable of protecting most of us most of the time. Lymphocytes derived from the thymus (T cells) or bone marrow (B cells) have the capacity to recognize foreignness when appropriately presented to them by specialized cells designed for that task. Recognition is followed by a veritable cascade of defensive responses, which work in concert to eliminate an invader. A pivotal T cell, which displays on its surface a differentiation antigen known as CD4, initiates any response by secreting, or causing to be secreted, a number of powerful cytokines, some of which promote directly the development of an inflammatory response, while others do so indirectly by passing inter-mediary and often permissive signals from one leukocyte to another. Such agents are referred to as interleukins, and 12 have been isolated at the time of writing. With the exception of those situations where organ-isms secrete a toxin, it is the release of cytokines and interleukins that produces the symptoms of infection, a fact relevant to the discussion below.

Within the T-cell system there are functionally distinct cells besides the CD4 inducer cell. Two are involved in an attack on an antigen, one cell producing the response referred to as delayed-type hypersensitivity (it takes 48 h for an optimal response to occur) and features specific T cells and macrophages. The other effector cell can physically bind to a cell infected by bacteria or viruses, as well as some tumor cells, and having done so, kill such cells. The fourth type of T cell is an immunoregulatory cell charged with monitoring and, if necessary, influencing the effector response to ensure that it is appropriate. An excessive undisciplined release of cytokines may produce unnecessary tissue damage.

All T cells recognize antigenic determinants via a receptor that has two chains projecting away from the surface of the cell, with a variable terminal region that has a specific three-dimensional configuration in space allowing one and only one antigenic determinant to have a best fit.

Bone marrow–derived B cells also recognize antigen, using a cell membrane-bound receptor for the purpose, but in this case the receptor is an immunoglobulin molecule (antibody) and it is immunoglobulins that are the secreted effector products of these cells. Antibodies are released once antigen is recognized by the B lymphocyte, and permission is provided from T cells, which allow for an optimum response.

By the time a human fetus is 16 weeks of age, T and B cells have been generated which can recognize more than a million different antigenic determinants, with any one cell being capable of recognizing only one of these determinants. In generating such diversity we may well be prepared for any encounter with foreignness, but the genetic permutations required generate cells capable of recognizing everything, including the proteins that constitute our own tissues. Hence there is a danger that such cells might initiate an attack on the self, damaging tissues or cells and producing an autoimmune disease.

PROTECTION FROM AUTOIMMUNE DISEASE

Relevant to our discussions are the extraordinary measures generated to overcome this potential problem. The ideal solution is simple enough: purge from the lymphocyte repertoire those cells capable of reacting to self. An attempt is made to do just that in the thymus, where many cells capable of recognizing our own individual antigen-presenting molecules are aborted by measures that are not fully understood. Similar, although less efficient, purging of cells that can recognize self occurs in the bone marrow. However, the system is imperfect and all of us are born with clones of cells capable of recognizing self that have escaped deletion and circulate in the blood and lymphatic vessels or reside in lymphoid tissues.

Post-thymic self-reactive T and B lymphocytes are a reality we have to live with throughout life. How are these cells prevented from engaging in autoaggressive maneuvers in most individuals? For tissue to be attacked, antigenic determinants of that tissue would need to be recognized by potentially autoaggressive T cells. This they can only do when antigen is presented as a complex, consisting of the antigen itself and one of four types of antigen-presenting molecules, easily recognized as products of the alleles existing at the A-, B-, C-, or D-locus on the short arm of chromosome 6 (human leukocyte antigens (HLA)). These proteins package, intracellularly, antigens for eventual display on a cell's surface in appropriately designed grooves. All cells display the A-, B-, and C-locus proteins on their surface and, theoretically at least, could present to T cells peptides derived from the cell, which would of course be 'self'. However, to initiate an immune response, the requirements are more restrictive. CD4 inducer lymphocytes only recognize antigenic determinants complexed to D-locus proteins, and these are not normally present on cells other than those specially designed to be antigen-presenting cells – usually macrophages. Thus, while cytotoxic T cells can attack antigen/A, B, or C complexes, they will only do so after permission has been given by CD4 lymphocytes, which will have recognized an antigen/D complex.

D-locus proteins can be generated on the surface of many cells which are normally not involved in antigen presentation when sufficient concentrations of a number of cytokines are released locally by the cells of the immune system itself. Viral infection in a tissue, for example, could generate, quite appropriately, the local release of interferon with an up-regulation of D-locus antigen expression on the infected cell (self) – a dangerous situation. Disciplined self-reactive lymphocytes must resist the temptation to attack in this circumstance. To help ensure that this occurs, at least two cooperative mechanisms are employed: antigen-specific suppressor T cells and anti-idiotypic antibodies.

Antigen-specific suppressor T cells can be activated by antigen to release specific molecules that suppress autoaggressive lymphocytes. Such cells monitor the appropriateness of immunological reactions. Of relevance to our discussion is the fact that the generation of anti-idiotypic antibodies facilitates such mechanisms, as well as providing an independent mechanism for 'neutralizing' autoantibodies.

Antibodies are composed of two heavy (long) and two light (short) chains of amino acids. The two heavy chains are held together by disulfide bridges, and at one end of the molecule the light chains are bound by a similar mechanism to the heavy chains. A molecule with a valency of two (two binding sites for antigen) is thus created. The three-dimensional shape in space created at the terminal end of the area where

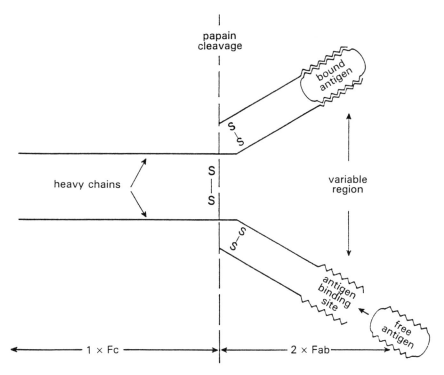

Figure 1 The basic anatomy of an immunoglobulin molecule. Two heavy and two light chains of amino acids are linked by disulfide (S–S) bridges. At one end of the molecule, a three-dimensional steric configuration (idiotypic determinant) of each arm allows one (and only one) antigenic determinant to enjoy 'best-fit' status. The molecule can be cleaved by digestion with papain. Two fractions that have antibody activity will be formed (Fab), and one fraction that tends to be relatively constant (Fc) will be formed. The amino acid sequence of the latter determines the major functional activity of the molecule. Reproduced with permission from Dwyer, J. M. (1987). Manipulating the immune system with intravenous immunoglobulin. *Adv. Intern. Med.*, **32**, 111–35

light and heavy chains fuse forms a binding site referred to as the idiotypic region, as it is specific for one antigenic determinant. The opposite end of the molecule consists of the terminal portions of the two heavy chains, and is referred to as the Fc portion of the molecule. The antigen-binding end of the molecule, i.e. the fraction with antibody activity, is referred to as the Fab region. The Fc portion of the molecule can bind certain complement proteins, and many cells have receptors for the Fc portion of an immunoglobulin as well as receptors for complement (Figure 1). It follows that patients with autoimmune diseases must have displayed D antigens on the surface of certain cells, and failed to suppress self-reactive T cells availing themselves of the opportunity presented by complexes of self attached to a D protein. Suppressor T cells and/or mechanisms involving anti-idiotypic regulatory molecules have failed to prevent an autoimmune response.

If autoreactive B cells, for one reason or another, produce autoantibodies to self tissue, they in turn generate the production of antibodies to determinants of themselves (antiantibodies). If the determinants involve structurally important areas of the binding site for antigen (the idiotypic region), then antibody to these sites would block the ability of the original antibody to bind to its antigen. The dimers so formed (antibody–antibody) will be removed by the cells of the reticuloendothelial system, following the binding of the complexes to receptors for the Fc portion of IgG found on the surface of such scavenger cells. Certain immunoregulatory T cells also have receptors for the Fc portion of IgG, and thus can bind IgG or complexes of idiotype and anti-idiotype. To understand the role of antibody in both the generation of and protection from autoantibodies, some anatomical features of such molecules need emphasizing.

B cells produce five classes of IgG, each being functionally specific as they expand our defensive repertoire. Of these molecules, IgG is the most important, and indeed life is not possible without its production. IgG is the main immunoglobulin component found in serum, and in most people the serum level of IgG is remarkably consistent. It seems most unlikely that serum levels merely represent the result of immunological activity occurring over the last few months (IgG has a half-life of approximately 26 days). It seems more likely that IgG is produced not just to counter foreign antigens, but for regulatory purposes as well. Such molecules may even exert an influence beyond the immune system itself. It is a common experience of clinical immunologists caring for patients with agammaglobulinemia to have them explain time and time again that they feel more mentally alert and perform better intellectually shortly after they have been given an infusion of immunoglobulin. Recent evidence suggests that all of us continuously produce small amounts of autoantibody, and thus we must constantly produce small amounts of anti-idiotypic antibody to neutralize any potential danger.

EFFECT OF IVIG ON AUTOIMMUNE DISEASES

In recent years, following the development of concentrated preparations of IgG that could be administered intravenously, it has become a matter of great interest to try and understand by what mechanism the infusion of large amounts of this product leads to the suppression of autoimmune phenomena. Immunoglobulin suitable for intravenous use (IVIG) was designed to facilitate replacement therapy for patients with a primary or secondary humoral immune deficiency state. It is now clear, however, that by rapidly increasing serum levels of IgG, the immune system can be manipulated by IVIG. Individual diseases shown to respond to IVIG are discussed below.

By what mechanisms could IVIG down-regulate the autoaggression of T and B lymphocytes? It has been noted that effective IVIG products contain high concentrations of dimers, i.e. IgG–IgG complexes. It has now been demonstrated that the presence of these dimers indicates the presence of significant concentrations of anti-idiotypic antibodies. It is likely that the major and sustaining influence of IVIG on autoimmune processes is mediated by a library of anti-idiotypic antibodies present in IVIG. Most manufacturers these days make their product from blood pooled from 10 000–20 000 donors, and thus have at their disposal an enormous repertoire of anti-idiotypic immunoglobulins, produced by so many different people challenged by so many different circumstances.

We now feel that many of the anti-idiotypic antibodies present in IVIG are capable of binding to low-affinity IgM autoantibodies produced by most of us most of the time. Such anti-idiotypic antibodies, and indeed such autoantibodies, are thought to play a relatively small role in the induction of any autoimmune phenomena. However, the production of high-affinity IgG 'renegade' autoantibodies capable of damaging, for example, red cells or platelets, require, for neutralization, anti-idiotypic antibodies not produced by normal healthy people. It appears that these regulatory anti-idiotypic antibodies are only found in significant concentrations in the plasma of individuals who are in remission from a disease featuring such autoantibodies, or are relatives of people who have produced such autoantibodies. It is likely in the latter situation that a genetic tendency favoring the production of autoimmune disease is only kept at bay by the production of these anti-idiotypic antibodies, which can bind to disease-producing autoantibodies. Because it has been demonstrated that a number of such anti-idiotypic antibodies can bind to the Fab region of autoantibodies against a number of self-determinants (e.g. DNA, thyroglobulin, factor VIII, etc.), broadly cross-reactive anti-idiotypic antibodies may be a feature of our normal immunoregulatory housekeeping when IgG autoantibodies appear.

Another demonstrable mechanism by which the IgG in IVIG can manipulate the immune response relates to the binding of IgG to Fc receptors on certain cells. If, for example, one had an autoimmune hemolytic anemia whereby antibody-coated red cells were being destroyed by cells of the reticuloendothelial system that bind to the Fc portion of the IgG bound to red cells, then saturating such receptors with IgG that is not bound to antigen, i.e. the IgG in IVIG, would have a protective effect. This has been clearly demonstrated to occur, as one can minimize the aggressive response to red cells coated with anti-D antibody by the prior infusion of IVIG.

It is possible, but has not been demonstrated, that antibodies in IVIG could clear from the circulation or a given tissue unidentified viruses that are perpetuating an immune response. It is also possible that IVIG down-regulates the production of Fc receptors on all cells, thus minimizing their opportunity to interact with autoantibodies, but the only immuno-manipulative mechanism thought to be of significance besides the production of anti-idiotypic antibody and the saturation of Fc receptors, involves the ability of IVIG to decrease the production of cytokines.

A number of disease processes are thought to be associated with an undisciplined and excessive release of cytokines. Such immuno-pathology is allergic in nature (allergy from the Greek for altered energy). We are more used to thinking in clinical medicine of allergic reactions occurring within the B-cell compartment (i.e. the production of excessive IgE), but we now know that the same phenomenon can affect T cells, and I am suggesting that we designate the type of allergy we are describing by the introduction into immunology of the terms 'tallergy' and 'ballergy'. Of great interest is that a number of those diseases thought to represent tallergy are down-regulated by the infusion of IVIG, e.g. Kawasaki syndrome, juvenile rheumatoid arthritis and chronic fatigue syndrome.

It is quite likely that a number of the mechanisms described above involve the activation of suppressor T cells and indeed, in a number of diseases, from myasthenia gravis to atopic eczema, it is possible to demonstrate increased and more appropriate immunoregulatory cell activity after the infusion of IVIG.

A recently recognized phenomenon in clinical immunology involves bacterial products referred to as super antigens. Staphylococci, streptococci and mycoplasma can produce molecules which, in genetically susceptible individuals, cause a tallergic response by binding to certain alleles in the variable region of the β-chain of the T-cell receptor. By bridging these receptors, they activate the T cell. Although the antigen-binding site of the T-cell receptor may be unique, a very large number of the T cells of any given individual will display the same allelic determinant, and thus it is possible for a super antigen to activate the majority of T lymphocytes in a susceptible individual. This can produce a fatal anaphylactic-like reaction, with the toxic shock syndrome being a classic example of the severity of the response that can be induced. It seems highly likely that IVIG can protect from such responses, although the mechanisms for this protection are as yet unclear.

CLINICAL EXPERIENCE WITH IVIG FOR IMMUNE MANIPULATION

IVIG therapy has been reported to be beneficial for more than 35 diseases thought to be produced by immunopathology. The published reports are listed in Tables 1, 2 and 3.

IVIG for immunohematological disorders

Immune thrombocytopenic purpura

Interest in the manipulative properties of IVIG on the immune system first developed with the report of a significant rise in the platelet count

Table 1 Intravenous immunoglobulin (IVIG) for immunohematological disorders

Disease	Comments
Thrombocytopenia	
Humoral deficiency and immune thrombocytopenic purpura	first descriptions included improvement in hemolytic anemia as well as immune thrombocytopenic purpura in immunodeficient children
Acute immune thrombocytopenic purpura in children	*see* text
Chronic immune thrombocytopenic purpura in children and adults	*see* text
Alloimmunization after platelet infusions, thrombocytopenia of pregnancy and neonatal thrombocytopenia	not autoimmune phenomena; normal response to histoincompatible platelets transfused or crossing maternal–fetal barriers; best results in intrauterine fetal thrombocytopenia (17 responses, 3 failures) and neonatal thrombocytopenia; in adults with thrombocytopenia after transfusions, results are variable; small double-blind placebo-controlled trial showed no significant sustained response
Gold-induced thrombocytopenia	one report; thrombocytopenia appears to be immunologically induced
Thrombotic thrombocytopenic purpura	three reports of variable but encouraging responses to IVIG with or without plasma exchange
Thrombocytopenia in hemolytic–uremic syndrome	response in eight children; suggested neutralization of bacterial toxin; only historic controls were used

continued

Table 1   (*continued*)

Disease	Comments
Anemia	
Autoimmune hemolytic anemia with or without immunodeficiency	variable results, no controlled trial; response more likely in patients with immunodeficiency
Autoimmune hemolytic anemia and immune thrombocytopenic purpura (Evan's syndrome)	one case only; good response
Red cell aplasia	may follow viral infection, often IgG and T–cell suppression of erythropoiesis demonstrable; treatment with Fab fragments successful? Provoking an anti–idiotypic response
Fetal–maternal Rh immunization	three cases, all treated during pregnancy; maternal anti-RhD suppressed
Neutropenia	
Autoimmune neutropenia	variable results but a number of good responses; no response in Felty's syndrome
Pure white cell aplasia	one case only with good response
Hemophilia A and B	
Associated with antibodies to factor VIII and IX	*see* text

Rh, rhesus

Table 2   Intravenous immunoglobulin (IVIG) for non-hematological auto-immune diseases

Disease	Comments
Myasthenia gravis	*see* text
Demyelinating polyneuropathy	*see* text
Guillain–Barré syndrome	autoantibodies to peripheral nerve myelin; 13 of 17 patients responded to 400 mg of IVIG/kg given over 5 days; multicenter controlled trial in progress
Multiple sclerosis	11 of 31 patients improved; condition stabilized in nine of 31 patients, but placebo was not given in this unblinded study
Systemic lupus erythematosus	hematological problems reversed in neonates whose mothers had systemic lupus erythematosus; maternal anticardiolipin antibodies blocked; better fetal survival; renal IgG deposits solubilized; too few cases for critical analysis
Polymyositis and Sjögren's syndrome	few cases of polymyositis treated, but substantial improvement noted in those few; IVIG reported to reduce steroid dependency in both conditions
Rheumatoid arthritis	seven of 10 patients responded to IVIG from human placentas; another study reported 50% improvement in 60% of 31 patients
Insulin-dependent diabetes mellitus	insulin dosage reduced in uncontrolled trial; controlled trial showed a trend towards reduction in insulin requirements at the end of 12 months
Bullous pemphigoid	autoantibodies to skin basement membrane; eight of 11 patients responded
Thyroid eye disease	eight patients responded after having no response to steroids, azathioprine, or both
Uveitis	one patient with severe uveitis; vitreous bleeding and opacities; no response to steroids, responded to IVIG; relapsed but responded to further IVIG

Table 3 Intravenous immunoglobulin (IVIG) for other diseases with immunopathology features

Disease	Comments
Kawasaki syndrome	*see* text
Chronic fatigue syndrome	humoral and cellular immune abnormalities; two controlled trials with different selection criteria and different instruments for assessment; significant improvement in one study, not confirmed by the other
Asthma in children	steroid-dependent, highly atopic children were given 2 g of IVIG/kg over 2 days; treated monthly for 6 months; skin-test and bronchial reactivity improved and steroid requirements reduced during controlled trial
Juvenile rheumatoid arthritis	dramatic effect on systemic symptoms, fever and rash; joints less responsive
Crohn's disease	12 patients treated in one study; ulcerative colitis responded better than Crohn's disease; other open studies yielded similar results
Recurrent abortions	no cardiolipin antibodies; five women who among them had lost 23 pregnancies were given 500 mg of IVIG/kg per month starting before conception; four had live-born infants and the 5th was well at 12 weeks of gestation
Graft-versus-host disease	apparent reduction noted during prophylaxis for infection
Human immunodeficiency virus infection in children	*see* text

in two patients with agammaglobulinemia and severe thrombocytopenia who received IVIG. This observation was soon complemented by reports that platelet counts in children with the Wiskott–Aldrich syndrome occasionally increased after IVIG (Table 1). Many studies of the efficacy of this treatment of acute immune thrombocytopenic purpura in children followed. So efficient has been IVIG for the management of this condition that it may be the therapy of choice for children with acute autoimmune thrombocytopenic purpura who need treatment.

Immune thrombocytopenic purpura in children and adults is associated with the presence in plasma and on platelets of antibodies to platelet glycoproteins IIb/IIIa and Ib/IX. An analysis of 28 published reports of the treatment of 282 children with this condition revealed an increase in the platelet count to more than $10 \times 10^9/l$ in 64%, and more than $50 \times 10^9/l$ in 83% of cases. In adults with immune thrombocytopenic purpura, treatment with IVIG in the first 6 months of the disease is more likely to produce long-term remission than treatment begun later. In children with immune thrombocytopenic purpura, if IVIG in a dose of $400\,mg\,kg^{-1}\,day^{-1}$ for 2 days induces a rise in the platelet count of $30 \times 10^9/l$ in the first 48 h of therapy, it is unlikely that further treatment will increase the therapeutic benefit. If there is not a satisfactory increase within 48 h, then a daily dose of 400 mg/kg should be given for 5 days.

Chronic immune thrombocytopenic purpura

The treatment with IVIG of children with chronic immune thrombocytopenic purpura has been almost as successful as that for acute immune thrombocytopenic purpura (62% have long-term improvement). Adults have responded less well, although the majority have had a substantial but short-lived increase in their platelet count. This transient increase may enhance the safety of splenectomy. In a recent study of nine adults with chronic immune thrombocytopenic purpura, all had serum antiplatelet antibodies directed against GPIIb/IIIa proteins that could be absorbed by IVIG. Treatment with $F(ab)_2$ fragments was also effective, suggesting that the inhibitory action of IVIG is mediated, at least in part, by the variable region of antibodies, probably by an anti-idiotypic mechanism. Such observations do not preclude the importance of Fc receptor blockade as an additional, and perhaps vital, component of the response.

Factor VIII and IX inhibitors

Inhibitors of antihemophilic factor (factor VIII) may cause a coagulopathy that is clinically similar to hemophilia. Such inhibitors may develop spontaneously in patients with autoimmune diseases, or after the administration of factor VIII. They are anti-factor VIII antibodies that occasionally react with factor IX as well. The levels of spontaneously appearing antibodies to factor VIII decreased within 36 h of the administration of IVIG, and in some patients secretion of anti-factor VIII antibodies was suppressed for 5 years. Evidence that the binding of $F(ab)_2$ fragments from the IVIG preparation to the autoantibody was responsible for the suppression provided the first convincing evidence for immunomanipulation by anti-idiotypic antibodies.

The development of antibodies to factors VIII and IX during treatment for hemophilia A or B is common, occurring in 8–20% of patients, and may be associated with episodes of uncontrollable bleeding. Tolerance to factors VIII and IX has been re-established using a combination of IVIG, the factors themselves, and cyclophosphamide. In 13 of 15 hemophiliac patients (11 with factor VIII deficiency and four with factor IX deficiency), this treatment eliminated the production of IgG4 antibodies to the crucial epitopes of the clotting factors. The mechanism is unknown, but tolerance cannot be achieved without the use of both IVIG and cyclophosphamide.

IVIG for non-hematological autoimmune diseases

Myasthenia gravis

Since 1982, more than 60 patients with myasthenia gravis have been treated with IVIG; clinical improvement has been noted in 73%. In two patients, treatment was associated with increased weakness. Myasthenia gravis is associated with the production of polyclonal antibodies to the 250 000-Da glycoprotein that acts as a receptor for acetylcholine at the neuromuscular junction. After IVIG therapy, the concentration of these antibodies decreased in 50% of patients. It is not clear, however, that this fall is the only, or indeed the major, mechanism responsible for the clinical response. Improvement may occur rapidly, sometimes within 24 h, and always within 3 weeks if the therapy is successful. The benefits have been reported to last for 40–90 days. In two reports, concurrent with improvement there was an increase in the number of circulating cells expressing the CD16 and CD8 differentiation antigens. Such cells may be natural killer cells or immunoregulatory cells. An increase in T lymphocytes expressing receptors for the Fc portion of IgG, which are also likely to be immunoregulatory cells, has also been noted. IVIG is not recommended as sole therapy for the management of myasthenia gravis, but it may allow a reduction in the dose of corticosteroids and immunosuppressive agents, and reduce symptoms during the months required for the latter therapies to become effective. Patients unresponsive to plasma exchange may benefit from IVIG. As with so many of the indications for IVIG, firm guidelines for its use in myasthenia gravis will require the performance of placebo-controlled studies.

Chronic inflammatory demyelinating polyneuropathy

Chronic inflammatory demyelinating polyneuropathy is the chronic form of Guillain–Barré syndrome, a problem from which 80% of patients make a satisfactory recovery in 6 months. In contradistinction to Guillian–Barré syndrome, such patients have more sensory changes and progressive weakness, but the respiratory muscles are involved less frequently, and the majority of patients have a poor prognosis. Their serum contains antibodies that react with myelin, Schwann cells and other nerve structures.

Several uncontrolled studies have reported improvement in patients with chronic inflammatory demyelinating polyneuropathy after treatment with IVIG. In one placebo-controlled crossover study, all seven patients who received IVIG (400 mg/kg for 5 days) improved, whereas there was no response to placebo in five patients. Nerve conduction velocities improved in only those patients who received IVIG. In a more extensive placebo-controlled trial involving 28 patients, the rates of response to placebo and IVIG were 23% and 26%, respectively. The rather high rate of response in the placebo-treated patients suggests that some patients had neuropathies other than chronic inflammatory demyelinating polyneuropathy. Analysis of the literature describing the use of IVIG in a total of 52 patients with chronic inflammatory demyelinating polyneuropathy suggests that a response to therapy is most likely if the disease has been present for less than a year, nerve conduction velocity in motor nerves is less than 80% of normal, and there is progressive rather than stable disease.

IVIG for other diseases featuring immunopathology

Kawasaki syndrome

Patients with the mucocutaneous lymph-node syndrome (Kawasaki disease), often have coronary artery disease. In a multicenter controlled trial of high-dose IVIG plus aspirin, compared with aspirin alone for the treatment of this condition, the IVIG regimen reduced the frequency of coronary artery abnormalities. These results were subsequently confirmed in another controlled American study. Although circulating immune complexes may be found in the serum of children with Kawasaki disease, the beneficial effects of IVIG are not associated with the disappearance of these complexes. It seems much more likely that this disease results from the excessive production of cytokines, and that the secretion or effects of such molecules are modified by IVIG. In these patients, neutralization of a bacterial toxin that may stimulate the release of cytokines in a manner analogous to that in the toxic shock syndrome, has been reported. The suppression of activated T cells in this condition, after IVIG treatment, has also been demonstrated.

It is fair to say that, as IVIG is an expensive product and relatively few controlled trials have been carried out, it is crucial for progress in this field to have protocols generated to facilitate the study of many of these diseases, using a multicentered approach, as many of the diseases under discussion are quite rare. Only when placebo-controlled trials have been completed will we be better able to delineate the protocols required to obtain the maximum benefit from IVIG. In the meantime, however, there is no doubt that many patients with autoimmune diseases are being helped by the administration of IVIG, and that it offers a therapeutic option in many a situation where alternative options are limited or even absent. Admittedly, it appears as though the administration of IVIG containing billions of different antibody molecules is a little like bringing every book in the library home to make sure that the one we really want is present. However, it is unlikely that in the near future molecular techniques will be able to supply us with monoclonal antibodies that will have the same effect as IVIG, for indeed it is the cocktail of immunological experiences represented in the pooled product that supplies us with such a powerful new therapeutic tool. Research must proceed apace if we are to better understand and better utilize such products.

21

Concluding remarks

A. Morell

Here in Mar del Plata we had the opportunity to share the experience of some of the most distinguished experts and scientists in the field of immunotherapy. It is my privilege to summarize some of the highlights of their presentations.

At the beginning, Dr Hässig reminded us of the fathers of prophylaxis and treatment with intravenous immunoglobulins (IVIGs), to whom he himself belongs. One of the principal observations made in the 1970s was the recognition of the two functional entities of the IgG molecule: the antigen recognition by Fab and the various effector functions mediated by the Fc moiety. This had an impact on the development of so-called native or unmodified IVIG preparations for clinical use.

We then learnt from Dr Cottier about the rationale of passive immunotherapy in the gut-associated toxic shock syndrome. The scenario of its development includes the role of the intestinal barrier failure. Polyspecific IVIG could be one means to counteract this situation, and has thus to be included in prophylactic and therapeutic strategies.

In his first presentation, Dr Rewald expressed fundamental philosophical thoughts on the immune system – using the term 'deterministic chaos' in this respect – which certainly needs much further consideration.

While the importance of the complement system as an effector and immune amplification mechanism is generally known, there is little evidence to date about how IVIG could prevent complement-induced damage in autoimmune disease. Dr Basta told us more about this type of immune modulation. His data in guinea pigs and in sera from patients suggest that high IgG levels induced with IVIG prevent C3 and C4 fragments from binding to target cells and inducing damage.

On the basis of his experience with IgG therapy in Rh hemolytic disease of the newborn, Dr Rewald proposed an interesting new action mechanism of IgG on the vascular endothelium by which leakage of erythrocytes from small vessels could be reduced.

The next speaker was Dr Dominioni. Many of us knew already of his elegant study demonstrating the survival benefit mediated by Sandoglobulin® (Sandoz) in septic shock. Everybody appreciated his interesting new findings on the influence of IVIG on phagocytic functions in these patients. The question raised here was: is this effect due to immunomodulation or to the classical opsonophagocytosis by specific antibodies or are there several mechanisms involved? This question was also pertinent for the following presentations: Dr Ramírez Osío and Dr Santos reviewed the important field of neonatal sepsis, discussing the pathogenetic mechanisms and the potentialities of IVIG in the prophylaxis and therapy. According to their experience, carefully selected septic newborns could benefit from IVIG. The last speaker of the Saturday morning session was Dr Caneiro-Sampaio. She reported appalling figures of acquired immune deficiency syndrome (AIDS) victims in Brazil and particularly of pediatric AIDS. In these functionally agammaglobulinemic children, the rationale for IVIG is prevention of pyrogenic infections, stabilization of T cells and suppression of autoimmune phenomena.

The first two presentations of the Saturday afternoon session were devoted to the modulation of the immune network with IVIG. Drs Kazatchkine and Kaveri introduced the principles of the concept of autoreactivity which is under tight control in health. Natural autoantibodies take part in a self-connected network of idiotype–anti-idiotype interactions. In patients with autoimmune disorders, this intrinsic network control is lost. As a consequence, disease-associated autoantibodies appear which either qualitatively or quantitatively differ from natural autoantibodies. The speakers then explained how natural autoantibodies present in IVIG – pooled from up to 16 000 plasma donations – can restore the functioning immune network in these patients. It is fascinating to observe how these investigators and their group constantly increase the body of evidence for this important mechanism of immunomodulation: IVIG presents not only a source of neutralizing autoantibodies, but also interacts with idiotypes on B and T lymphocytes.

Dr Leal, as the last speaker of the day, gave us a very valuable critical review of the use of intravenous immunoglobulin (IVIG) in severe pediatric diseases caused by viruses. He discussed the pros and cons of IVIG in these conditions, and added many case reports demonstrating his personal experience in the field. Again, the fundamental question is whether IVIG should contain large amounts of virus-specific neutralizing antibodies or whether the beneficial action is mediated by not yet defined immunomodulatory mechanisms.

In the Sunday morning session we listened to Drs Newland and Imbach, who have gathered more than a decade of experience on IVIG treatment of immune thrombocytopenia in adults and children. As you all know, what is now termed 'immunomodulation' started with their work on idiopathic thrombocytopenic purpura (ITP), and we are proud at the Swiss Red Cross that this work was done with Sandoglobulin. Both speakers concentrated on mechanisms of action of IVIG. There is a clear difference between immediate effects mediated by Fc receptor blockade and late or long-term effects.

A fascinating presentation was given by Dr Coulam. Evidence is rapidly growing for a benefit of Sandoglobulin® (Sandoz) in recurrent spontaneous abortion. Demonstration of the effect in each patient, be it success or failure, necessitates thorough clinical investigation. Her hypothesis of the pathogenesis of immune-mediated recurrent spontaneous abortion, an idiotype–anti-idiotype mechanism, still needs further substantiation.

Dr Bullorsky, presenting on behalf of Professor Boogaerts, summarized the rationale of IVIG therapy in bone marrow transplantation. In some countries, allogeneic bone marrow transplantation has evolved into one of the most important applications of IVIG. Here again, we are faced with the question of antibody titers, most notably anti-cytomegalovirus (CMV) titers in IVIG. It is not yet clear how prevention of CMV disease by IVIG relates to its immunomodulatory activity in acute graft-versus-host disease.

Dr Benaim presented us with an impressive series of slides on severe burns patients. Defense mechanisms are evidently disturbed in a multifaceted way in such patients. Accordingly, treatment is very complex, and replacement of IVIG can correct only one of the many factors that are damaged or missing.

Dr González Martín introduced juvenile rheumatoid arthritis to the audience. His clinical trial shows that IVIG has an impact on peripheral T-cell subsets. In children who responded favorably to treatment, the CD4 : CD8 ratio increased due to a fall in the CD8 subset.

In the afternoon, Dr Gelfand discussed the topic of specific antibodies versus immunomodulation with IVIG using the example of patients with congenital antibody deficiencies. It becomes increasingly clear that, in these patients as well as in autoimmune and inflammatory diseases, immunomodulation and anti-inflammatory effects of IVIG are of upmost importance. Asthma therapy is another condition where IVIG can exert an anti-inflammatory activity. I think it was Dr Gelfand who coined the term 'steroid-sparing' effects of IgG (summarized in Dr Rewald's review), which is clinically so relevant in many of the disease states mentioned during this Symposium.

Finally, Dr Borberg informed us about important new developments in the treatment of autoimmune diseases. He uses plasma exchange therapy to remove pathogenic auto-antibodies or circulating immune complexes, a procedure that can be combined or followed by application of IVIG for immunomodulation.

An even more sophisticated approach seems to be immune apheresis using anti-IgG or other immunoadsorbent columns which can also be followed by IVIG treatment. Preliminary evidence shows that this combined treatment opens new avenues in the therapy of autoimmune disorders.

How can we now sum up this wealth of information in a few words? First, we have gained an excellent overview of disease states in which intravenous immunoglobulins have an immunomodulatory activity without neglecting opsonophagocytosis. Second, because most speakers devoted time to the pathogenesis and to the mechanisms of action, we now understand much better the term 'immunomodulation by IVIG', a phrase which previously was rather nebulous. It includes blockade of cellular receptors, network interactions by idiotypes/anti-idiotypes, and of course also anti-inflammatory activities by interference with the cytokine cascade.

Index